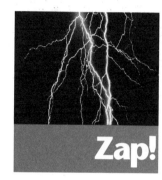

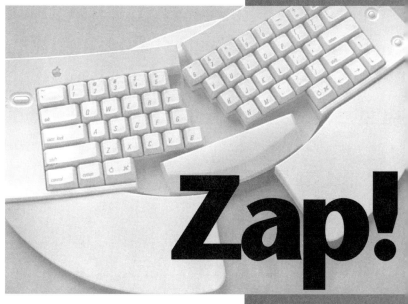

# Zap!

**How your computer can hurt you—and what you can do about it**

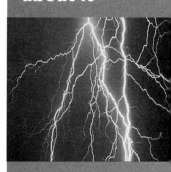

## by Don Sellers

Edited by Stephen F. Roth

PEACHPIT PRESS    AN OPEN HOUSE BOOK

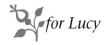 *for Lucy*

ZAP! How your computer can hurt you—and what you can do about it
Don Sellers
Edited by Stephen F. Roth

PEACHPIT PRESS, INC.
2414 Sixth St.
Berkeley, CA 94710
510/548-4393
510/548-5991 (fax)

LIBRARY OF CONGRESS CATALOGING-IN-PUBLICATION DATA
Sellers, Don.
  Zap! : how your computer can hurt you and what you can do about it / by Don Sellers : edited by Stephen F. Roth.
      p.    cm.
  "An Open House book."
  Includes index.
  ISBN 1-56609-021-0
  1. Human-computer interaction. 2. Human engineering. 3. Computers--Health aspects. I. Roth, Stephen F., 1958-
  II. Title.
  QA76.9.H85S45  1994      613.6'2--dc20      93-46277
0 9 8 7 6 5 4 3 2

Printed and bound in the United States of America

Printed on recycled paper.

# Contents

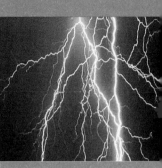

JUN - 1996

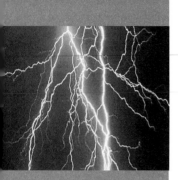

# Preface

## A Handbook for Safer Computing

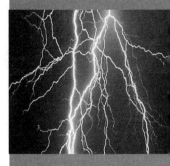

"What's wrong?"

"My wrists are killing me. They've hurt off and on for years, but not bad enough to see my doctor. A few months ago I had a big project with a really killer deadline. My wrists began aching, but I kept going, figuring it would pass. They haven't stopped hurting since."

"Can't the doctor do anything?"

"He told me to wear these splints and take aspirin when it hurt too much. He suggested surgery, but I'm not sure I want that."

"Can't you see another doctor?"

"Who?"

"Isn't there another way to treat this?"

My friend was completely transformed from when I had seen her only a few months earlier. Suffering chronic pain, she could only put in a few hours a day at her freelance job. Gardening, which she loved, proved impossible. With her livelihood threatened, she was near despair.

How did she get into this mess? Was her desk the wrong height? Were her work habits wrong? Did she get too little exercise? Or too much? Had this problem been creeping up on her for years, without her knowing? Was her problem preventable? How many others were at risk? Could it happen to me?

## The Cost of Computer Injury

My friend was not alone—the number of people suffering computer-related injuries has risen dramatically with the popularity of desktop computers. The Bureau of Labor Statistics (BLS) surveys show that in 1981, when the desktop computer was just being introduced, cumulative trauma disorders (CTDs) affected 23,000 workers, accounting for 18 percent of all workplace illnesses in the United States (this includes all industries, like meatpacking and

*Many computer-related injuries are preventable.*

■■■
**Use common sense.**
■■■

vii

working in a supermarket). By 1992, when there were over 50 million desktop computers in use, the number had risen to 281,800, or 62 percent.

While the BLS percentages may accurately reflect the accelerated injury rate, the actual numbers of those considered injured by the BLS are commonly held to be significantly understated. Recently, a *CTDNews* survey concluded that 4.4 million people in the United States suffer from computer-related CTDs alone.

No one knows how much this costs businesses, but most rough estimates place it in the tens of billions of dollars. The National Council on Compensation Insurance figures that treating a single case of back pain costs business about $24,000; treating a single case of carpal tunnel syndrome costs $29,000. Not all those suffering from computer-related CTDs have sought treatment; if they did, the cost to business could reach upwards of $100 billion dollars a year. Better surveys must be made before the real figures are known.

## *Zap!* Fights Back

I wrote *Zap!* because I knew this near-epidemic could be reversed—with education and effort. *Zap!* acts as a handbook that sifts the fact from the fancy of computer health issues by providing answers to the most commonly asked questions about computer health.

**Can you get injured by working on a computer?** Yes.

**Are you likely to?** Probably not, depending on your job type, equipment, schedule, body, and stress level.

**Do computer injuries debilitate people?** Yes, a small minority.

**Can injury be prevented?** In many cases, yes.

Most computer users don't know what can injure them. And people often work on computers until their body is so injured that a return to good health proves difficult or impossible. *Zap!* explains the steps to take to minimize the chances that your computer will hurt you. *Zap!*'s mission is simple: reduce the number of people who are ever injured by a computer to a minimum.

## How to Read This Book

Steve Roth, my editor, has a sign above his desk that reads "Eschew Obfuscation," and we tried to carry that simple philosophy to *Zap!*: most chapters describe problems, then supply ways you can prevent and fix them. For you to get the most out of this book, think of it as one of the tools at your disposal: *Zap!* supplies the information, but you must add your own intelligence and common sense. *Zap!* can guide you, but it cannot necessarily tell you exactly what you should do in any particular situation. You may need to go beyond *Zap!*, seeking the advice of a professional, for example, in order to use a computer safely. Here's how to work with *Zap!*.

### Don't Let It Replace a Doctor

To make *Zap!* useful for the largest number of people, I have included more information than most people need—so much, in fact, that you may have to steer clear of some. For example, I've included exercises and stretches in *Zap!*. Should everyone do them? Absolutely not (for example, you many not be healthy enough to engage in vigorous exercise). *Zap!* also relates how certain medical conditions are typically handled. Should you handle them that way? Perhaps. Only a health-care professional, and ultimately a physician, can tell you what is best for your body. Although I interviewed dozens of physicians, scientists, ergonomists, and other experts in the fields related to computer health, no book is capable of acting as a health-care professional.

> ■■■
> **Worry is counter-productive.**
> ■■■

### Be a Low-Stress Reader

*Zap!*'s tone expresses a reasoned concern about computer-health issues—far from the hysteria sometimes found in the general and computer press. There's a good reason for this choice: Psychological stress exacerbates most of the physical problems associated with computer use. Worry is counterproductive. Read *Zap!* with a positive attitude, figure out what you need to do, and then take action.

### Keep Informed of Current Events

The computer health field excites scientists because it is changing so rapidly. While most of the information in *Zap!* will be accurate for quite some time, it's impossible to predict what will change, and how. Keep yourself current on the subject through newspapers and computer magazines. And I'll bring out revised editions when necessary.

## Acknowledgments

The thinness of *Zap!* belies the great number of people who contributed to its content. I thank them all for helping to create a handbook for safer computing.

### Kate Rauch

Kate Rauch contributed her broad expertise as a health journalist to write several chapters of *Zap!*. Her knowledge and judgment contributed greatly to the success of this book. I am fortunate to have had her help.

## Computer Health Experts

Creating *Zap!* required the insights of scores of computer health experts. Their selfless generosity with their time and knowledge is a testament to their dedication both to this subject and to their particular fields and organizations. The following people were interviewed to ensure the content of *Zap!* is factual, comprehensive, and up to date.

Bruce Bernard, MD, MPH, National Institute of Occupational Safety and Health (NIOSH); Robert Bettendorf, Institute for Office Ergonomics; Mark Caitlin, WASHCOSH; Richard Cheu, Vision Aerobics; Elizabeth Collumb, Voyager Company; Paul Cornell, PhD, Steelcase, Inc.; Andrea Devaux, American Academy of Ophthalmology; Janet Gold, Labor Occupational Health Center; Fred Frietag, BO, Diamond Headache Clinic; Michelle Hartzell, NoRad Corporation; Rob Henning, PhD, University of Connecticut; Pamela Henwood, Visionary Software; Peter Jeff, Steelcase, Inc.; Pete Johnson, Ergonomics Laboratory at University of California at Berkeley and San Francisco; Marilyn Joyce, The Joyce Institute; Jim Kinsella, *CTDNews*; Rani Lueder, Humanics; Shirley Lunde, Kinesis Corporation; Steve Marshall, The Ergonomics Lab; Bob Matthews, Sonera Technologies; Dennis McIntosh, Center for Office Technology; Stephen C. Miller, OD, American Optometric Association; Lori Parent, Curtis Manufacturing; Vern Putz-Anderson, PhD, NIOSH; Ward Raap, National EMF Testing Association; David Rempel, MD, Ergonomics Laboratory at University of California at Berkeley and San Francisco; Caroline Rose, RSI Network; Hector Serber, American Ergonomics Corporation; Michael Silva, Enertech Consultants; Michael J. Smith, PhD, Department of Industrial Engineering, University of Wisconsin at Madison; Laura Stock, Labor Occupational Health Program; Suzanne Stefanac; Debbie Stiles, MN, RN, Healthy Dimensions; Naomi Swanson, PhD, NIOSH; Susan Thomas, Signa Corporation; Beverley Tillery, Office Technology Education Project; Ignacio Valdes, LifeTime Software; Thomas van Overbeek, Cornerstone Technology; Tim Warner, *Macworld* Magazine; Jim Young, NYCOSH.

And a special thanks to Dennis Ankrum, Human Factors Analyst, Nova Office Furniture; Mary Flynn, OD, Illinois College of Optometry; Chris Grant, PhD, University of Michigan; Ruth Lowengart, MD, Alta Bates Occupational Health Clinic; Dr. James Sheedy, VDT Eye Clinic, University of California; and Louis Slesin, *VDT NEWS*.

## Bookmakers

All books require the expertise of the behind-the-scenes experts in editorial and publishing to take a sprawling, meandering text and shape it into a cogent and tidy whole. I thank my experts for their contributions that molded *Zap!*.

Steve Roth, master of the art of editing, gave his perspicacity and advocacy; Ted Nace, Peachpit's ardent publisher, tirelessly husbanded this project through many incarnations; Olav Martin Kvern, guru-to-the-mavens, created the exquisite design and supplied continual support; Sandy Haight, talented artist (and old friend), produced the perfect illustrations; Glenn Fleishman, jack-of-all-trades, excelled as editor, fact checker, production manager, illustration coordinator, and reality touchstone; David Blatner, alternate reality touchstone, contributed his wisdom and insight.

**The Others**
I can never adequately thank my family for the long hours I spent away from them while I was researching and writing *Zap!*. Finally, I want to thank the many sufferers of computer injuries who so willingly shared their knowledge and lives with me. I hope this book helps.

Don Sellers

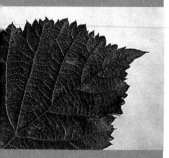

# 1 Introduction

## Office Ecology

*You and your office environment form one organic unit.*

■ ■ ■

**Changes in one aspect of the office environment can affect many others.**

■ ■ ■

It may seem odd to regard your office as an ecosystem, but it is. Your workplace environment holds living, breathing organisms— you and your co-workers. The quality of your health results from a delicate balance between what you bring with you to the office (how much you exercise, what you ate the night before, your outlook on life), the physical characteristics of the office (lighting, furniture, quality of the air), the requirements of your job (intensity of your keyboard use, amount of work rotation), and the psycho-social aspects of the workplace (deadlines, attitude of your manager, the emphasis your company puts on health). A combination of these factors affects whether you will be healthy or whether you will be injured, and to what extent.

## An Ecosystem in Trouble

The office ecosystem is under pressure: the downsizing of many businesses, management's expectation for increased productivity, inadequately designed equipment and furniture, and the rise in computer use have all contributed to the stress. That stress injures people. Computer-related injuries exact a high cost to employers and society due to medical treatment, lost wages, lost productivity, and retraining of disabled workers.

These injuries—most commonly involving the hands, wrists, arms, neck, and back—can be debilitating. The earlier they are diagnosed and correctly treated, the more likely that the injured person can be helped.

### It's All Hooked Together

The interdependent nature of different elements in the office ecosystem makes intervention a challenge. When you act to achieve safety at your computer, you often discover that a change in one component affects others. For example, you can't see the

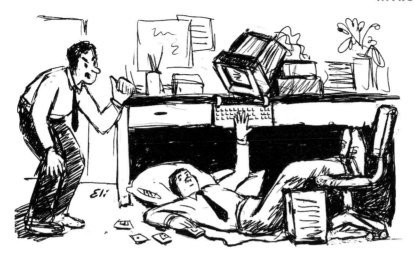

"Ergonomically correct or not, get up and look busy."

characters on your screen, so you pull the monitor closer. But then your neck hurts because you are bending it at too great an angle. Or you may find that your neck pain has nothing to do with your workstation or posture, but results from high levels of anxiety in your office. A useful solution can be elusive, because it must result from a knowledge and respect for the entire office ecosystem. All aspects of the office must exist in harmony to minimize stress on its most important inhabitant: you.

### Dangers of Delay

Like a natural ecosystem, when something goes out of whack in the office, it might not be immediately obvious. Your body and your mind usually compensate, minimizing the immediate effect. People adjust to constrained positions, chairs at the wrong height, and bosses who put them in lousy moods. But when the adjustment becomes chronic, the body becomes ripe for injury. Most computer-related injuries result from the accumulation of repeated stresses and minor injuries. The trick to working safely in the office ecosystem is ensuring that no factor in the environment puts undue stress on your body or your mind. You must be comfortable—physically and mentally—to ensure good health.

### Prevention and Early Intervention

As the ad says: You can pay me now or pay me later. The longer computer-related injuries are ignored, the more difficult it is to fix them. Letting a bad situation go on for too long can lead to permanent disability. Don't let it happen to you. Prevention and early

> ■ ■ ■
> **Safe computing results from an attitude of working with the environment.**
> ■ ■ ■

## Let the Buyer Beware

There's a lot of ergonomically design-ed hardware on the market, but just because something is labeled ergo-nomic doesn't mean that it is. The American National Standards Institute (ANSI) publishes specifications for computer workstations and the US Occupational Safety and Health Ad-ministration (OSHA) issues some recommendations, but neither orga-nization has a certification process to determine whether a product actually conforms to them. Beware of unsupported claims.

intervention (both medical treatment and modifica-tion of the workplace and job) are the keys to reduc-ing computer-health problems. Listen to your body; when something hurts, intervene in a constructive way. If you don't take the time to be healthy now, you may have to take the time to be sick later.

## Paths to Injury

To successfully modify the office ecosystem, it helps to understand the major factors that can lead to injury: the physical office environment, physical de-mands of the job, and psychological atmosphere of the workplace. What you bring to the workplace can also play a role—such as your reaction to de-manding situations or whether you have any pre-existing injuries.

### Office Environment

When you suspect you are being injured, the natural first reaction is to blame the physical environment. It's also the first place people tend to make changes. That reaction can be appropriate, but only if you modify the workplace correctly.

Your wrists hurt? The knee-jerk reaction is often: Get a wrist rest; in fact, get wrist rests for the entire department. That solution may succeed for some em-ployees; good ergonomics (the field of designing a physical environment that provides the proper fit for your body) is necessary to ensure safety. But ergo-nomic soundness is achieved by how the equipment is used, as well as how the equipment is designed and fits the individual. The physical aspects of your of-fice—chair, desk, lights, and so forth—are merely some of the tools you must use to work safely.

### Requirements of the Job

Many computer jobs have inherent dangers. Repeti-tive actions like typing on a keyboard can lead to cu-mulative trauma disorders. Many computer users type with too much force, which also puts them at risk for injury. With the push from management for more productivity, especially from the computer worker, the intensity of computer use has increased, and so have computer-related injuries. However, ergonomists have seen that interspersing computer work with other work can increase productivity.

### Psychosocial Aspects of the Workplace

Researchers have discovered that psychological stress plays a role in many workplace illnesses. Some researchers feel it is *the most important* cause. Many computerized offices have a deadline-oriented atmosphere and although such office stress can be a positive force for productivity, too much psychological stress increases muscle tension and makes it difficult for the body to function naturally. Many organizations are realizing that it is in their best interests to decrease pressure. Smart work organization—including giving employees a voice in the design of their work tasks—reduces psychological stress.

### What You Bring with You

The most often overlooked aspect of the office ecosystem is what you bring with you. Preexisting conditions, whether outright injuries or overuse of parts of your body, can play a significant role in CTDs. Hobbies such as gardening or playing the violin are known to exacerbate certain types of CTDs. Your physiology, habits, and attitudes—how heavy or thin you are, how you sit, how engrossed you can become in your work, and how you react to anxiety-producing situations—can also be a factor.

## The Safer Attitude

Reducing global pollution requires a fundamental shift in most people's behavior. Minimizing stress—both psychological and physical—in the office ecosystem requires an equally fundamental shift. Although quick fixes can be effective, the long-term solution to reducing stress on the entire system requires that you get an attitude.

The "safer computing" attitude requires you to act constructively *before* you feel the pain. Better

## One Priority

The trend at many companies in recent years has been to reduce mobility of the worker—put the computer user in a chair and leave him or her there all day long. That's wrong. If you could only do one thing to make yourself safer at the computer it should be: *move.*

The human body is not designed for sitting for long periods. Shifting position in your chair rotates stress between different muscle groups, allowing some to rest and recuperate, while others work. Getting up and walking down the hall relaxes your hands, wrists, arms, back, neck, eyes, and mind. Taking breaks increases productivity. Get up and go.

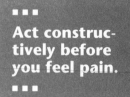

**Act construc-
tively before
you feel pain.**

health pays benefits throughout the organization. One after another, major corporations have begun to nurture this attitude in
their employees, making office safety a top priority, because it is in
their best interests to do so.

An OSHA ergonomist predicted recently that unless something
changes, by the turn of the century, one half of all business medical costs will go to treat cumulative trauma disorders. That trend
can be reversed if enough people adopt the safer computing attitude. But even one person can make a big difference.

**6**

# Eyestrain 2

## The Most Common Complaint

If you use a computer, the odds are that you've had eye discomfort. Eyestrain is the most common health complaint from computer users: 10 million cases of computer-related eyestrain are seen by optometrists every year. The following conditions increase your risk of eyestrain.

■ Intensive use. The more time spent on a computer, the greater the risk of straining your eyes.

■ Inadequate or detrimental lighting and monitor conditions.

■ Preexisting eye conditions, including those you may not be aware of.

■ Stress.

## Anatomy of Eyestrain

In nearly all cases, the cause of eyestrain is simple: trying to see under adverse conditions. The operation of your eyes is controlled by muscles, and, like any muscles, they can tire. If you're an average computer user, seeing is usually effortless; you don't realize it, but each day your eyes make approximately 30,000 movements. Your eye muscles do it automatically—scan a page, flip up to your monitor, refocus, glance at the clock, refocus again, and then jump back to your monitor. But it is muscular work.

A typical scenario places you in front of the computer, under a deadline. The banks of overhead fluorescents are too bright and your screen is fogged by their reflections. You concentrate for long periods on the screen and then rapidly shift focus from the screen to the reading material by your keyboard. Either holding a static position or rapidly moving your eyes can fatigue some of your eye muscles—the directional control muscles and possibly the ciliary muscles (which control the flexing of the crystalline lens

*As many as 40 percent of intensive computer users experience eyestrain.*

■■■

**Adverse conditions set the stage for eyestrain.**

■■■

## Related chapters:

■ Glasses and Contact Lenses

■ Lighting

■ Monitors

■ Stress

# The Many Forms of Eyestrain

*Eyestrain is an inexact term that's associated with various symptoms. Warning: Some of these symptoms can be caused by a much more serious condition or disease. Do not hesitate to seek the counsel of an optometrist or ophthalmologist.*

**Color perception.** *When you stare at a screen for long periods, especially one displaying green characters on a dark background, you can have difficulty perceiving colors properly when you look away. This phenomenon (called the McCulloch afterimage) occurs because of depletion of color-specific chemicals in the retina. However, your eye soon regenerates the lacking chemicals and the problem disappears.*

**Double vision.** *The convergence-control muscles allow both of your eyes to point at something near you. When they tire, double vision can occur—especially if you already have a marginal problem in keeping your eyes aligned. Fatigue in the convergence system is often not perceived directly, but rather felt as a headache or generalized fatigue. Double vision can also be the symptom of serious health problems; if the condition appears suddenly or persists, see an eye-care professional.*

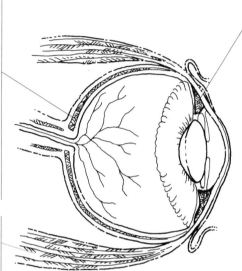

**Focusing problems.** *The most common symptom of eyestrain is impairment of your focusing ability, but how this happens isn't precisely known. Some experts believe that overworking the ciliary muscles by repeatedly shifting focus (for example between your keyboard and screen), or holding the same focus for too long, causes them to tire and lose their responsiveness.*

**Headaches.** *When you are under stress or sit motionless for long periods in front of a computer, you can get headaches. Most computer-related headaches are tension headaches, caused by muscle tension in the neck and head area and often generalized all over the head. These headaches are not caused directly by eyestrain but result from the accompanying effort of trying to see in poor conditions, or from compensating for inadequate eyesight by maintaining an awkward body position—for example, by tilting the head to see through bifocals. See* **Headaches.**

that allows you to change the distance at which your eyes focus). Your eyes no longer focus easily; you feel a headache coming on. You have eyestrain.

## Preventing and Relieving Eyestrain

You can help prevent eyestrain by changing your schedule, your environment, and perhaps having an eye examination.

## Refocus

Dr. Jim Sheedy of Berkeley's VDT Eye Clinic encourages computer users to look up from the computer every 10 minutes or so and refocus as far as possible into the distance for five or 10 seconds. The problem is getting people to remember to do it. Hint: many macro programs can trigger a time-dependent alarm. See **Software**.

## Give Your Eyes a Break

Take breaks or reschedule your work to allow different visual tasks. The National Institute of Occupational Safety and Health (NIOSH) recommends a rest break of 15 minutes for every two hours of moderately demanding VDT work, and a 15-minute break for every hour of intensive VDT use. Some experts suggest also taking frequent mini-breaks. What to do while taking breaks?

**Get away from it all.** When you leave your workstation and move to another location during a rest break, you lessen the muscular load on both your eyes and body, and have an opportunity to interact with others. Bonus: Rest breaks are known to have a beneficial effect on overall job performance. See **Schedules**.

**Get noncomputer work done.** Many people find they can schedule their noncomputer work as breaks away from their computer throughout the day, minimizing eye problems.

## Relax

Since psychological stress exacerbates eye stress, use breaks as a time to practice stress-reduction techniques. In his book *20/20—A Total Guide to Improving Your Vision and Preventing Eye Disease,* Dr. Mitchell Friedlaender recommends, "Stop using your eyes. Put your head back and your feet up and close your eyes for a few moments. Dim the lights. Put a damp washcloth over your eyes. Relax. And don't worry about it." This advice may be tough to follow in a busy office, so be resourceful; relax any way you can. See **Stress**.

## Will I Permanently Damage or Alter My Eyesight Using Computers?

There is controversy. Many vision experts don't believe you can permanently damage your eyesight using computers. The American Academy of Ophthalmology states that video display terminals (VDTs) present no hazard to the eye. A number of studies have shown that the eyes of computer users do not change significantly as compared to control groups of noncomputer users.

Other experts, including Dr. James Sheedy, chief of Berkeley's well-respected VDT Eye Clinic, say that while it's largely true that people can't injure their eyes at the computer, there is reason to believe physiological changes may occur in the eyes as a result of working on a computer or with any close object. Evidence indicates that extended near work may cause adult onset of myopia (nearsightedness). "It was considered a fringe idea five years ago that myopia could be caused by the environment or work habits," Sheedy states. "The scientific community is now ahead of the clinical community in the belief that there can be an environmentally caused myopia."

## Eyestrain Alert

Do you find the eye problems you suffer all week miraculously disappear over the weekend? Such a recurring pattern indicates computer-caused eyestrain. And don't be fooled: sometimes neck, back, or shoulder pain is actually the result of an awkward posture caused by straining to see.

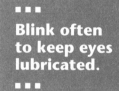

Blink often to keep eyes lubricated.

### Control the Lights and Monitor

Controlling the lighting in your work environment often alleviates eyestrain. Glare, reflection, high ambient light, and inadequately illuminated reading material are often the culprits. You must ensure that your monitor is adjusted properly and the screen is clean. See **Lighting** and **Monitors.**

### Modify the Work Area

Shifting between reading material and screen can cause eyestrain, especially if they are at extremely different distances from your eyes. Experts usually suggest that you place printed materials on a clip or copy stand adjacent to the monitor, although one recent study showed no increase in eyestrain when these materials were at different distances. Position the monitor 18 or more inches from your eyes (assuming you have adequate correction), and at a downward gaze angle. Traditional advice placed the top of the screen between eye level and 15 degrees below eye level, but some experts suggest lower may be better. See **Monitors.**

### Get an Eye Exam

Anyone beginning work on a VDT should get an eye examination from an eye doctor who understands VDT problems, and each year seek a follow-up exam. Sight sufficient for other tasks often doesn't stand up to the demands and unique working distance of computer work—until the eyesight is adequately corrected. Eyes change over time; an eye exam will detect any problems. See **Glasses and Contact Lenses.**

## Dry Eyes

Dry eyes—often associated with computer work—are caused by a lack of lubricating tears. Dry eyes can worsen and cause eyestrain; the condition is particularly onerous to contact lens wearers, and can be brought on by a number of factors.

**Staring.** People blink considerably less when they are using computers, so tears—your eyes' natural lubricant—aren't spread over the eye surface properly. Additionally, if you stare at an object high in your visual field—where most peoples' monitors are located—you open the eyelids more, resulting in increased tear evaporation.

**Lack of moisture in the air.** Many office buildings have dry atmospheres. The heat generated by your computer can also dry out the air. Both of these factors can increase tear evaporation from the eye. See **Office Air.**

**Medications.** Many medications, such as diuretics and antihistamines, can reduce the production of lubricating tears. See a pharmacist or the doctor who prescribed the medication to see if it is causing your dry eyes.

**Aging.** As you age, your body's tear production decreases, a problem suffered particularly by women over the age of 40 (see *The Aging Eye*, page 16).

### Solutions for Dry Eyes

Over-the-counter eye drops are a quick remedy for dry eyes. If you use eye drops, get those that are just lubricants, based on methyl cellulose or polyvinyl alcohol. Eye drops containing decongestants or vasoconstrictors can result in a rebound effect, actually causing the eye to dry. Whether or not you use eye drops, blink often—at least every five seconds—to keep eyes properly lubricated. Also, lowering your monitor will expose less of the eye's surface and reduce tear evaporation.

## Resources

See **Where Else to Turn** for a complete list of companies, products, associations, and other helpful resources.

*20/20: A Total Guide to Improving Your Vision and Preventing Eye Disease*, Mitchell H. Friedlaender and Stef Donvev (Emmaus, Pennsylvania: Rodale Press, 1991).

**American Academy of Ophthalmology**, PO Box 7424, San Francisco, CA 94120-7424. (415) 561-8500.

**American Optometric Association**, 243 North Lindbergh Blvd., St. Louis, MO 63141. (314) 991-4100.

## Vision Aerobics

Vision Aerobics, a unique software package designed to relieve eyestrain, uses arcade-style games for exercising the eyes during prolonged stints at the computer. In fact, its authors claim that Vision Aerobics goes beyond simple eyestrain relief, enhancing visual performance, reading speed, and hand-eye coordination. See **Software**.

# 3 Glasses and Contact Lenses

**Correcting Your Vision for Computer Use**

*Thirty percent of working-age Americans suffer from uncorrected or inadequately corrected vision problems.*

■ ■ ■

**Computer work demands sharp vision.**

■ ■ ■

What's going on? You can see the road clearly when you're driving, and your TV looks sharp, but your computer screen seems fuzzy. Or, perhaps, since you bought new bifocals, sitting at the computer produces neckaches. You're not alone: millions of computer users suffer distress due to preexisting eye conditions for two major reasons.

■ Computer work is particularly demanding on the eyes. An inadequacy in your visual system—even if you aren't aware of it—makes it difficult to see a computer screen clearly.

■ Many forms of eyesight correction cause rather than correct problems at the computer. Computer work may require custom eyesight correction.

Because eyesight degrades with age, almost all computer users will eventually need to address the issue of the quality of their eyesight and how best to correct it. Having glasses or contact lenses with the proper prescription is integral to achieving visual comfort for millions of computer users.

## Do You Need Glasses?

Uncorrected vision problems are widespread; 30 percent of working-age people in the United States have an uncorrected or inadequately corrected vision problem.

### Demanding Work

Working at a computer places demands on the eyes which the rest of everyday behavior does not. Healthy, adequately corrected eyes may be able to cope with these demands without suffering problems, whereas inadequately corrected eyes might not.

**Related chapters:**

■ Eyestrain

■ Lighting

■ Monitors

# Common Eye Problems

*Most glasses and contact lenses are
prescribed for a few different eye problems.*

**Myopia.** *Myopics cannot bring objects at a distance into focus,
but can focus on objects that are closer—sometimes, in extreme
cases, only those that are very close. People with a small
amount of myopia may be able to take off their glasses and
work comfortably at the computer. When those with more pro-
nounced myopia do the same, they often move too close to the
screen, and postural problems can result.*

**Hyperopia.** *Hyperopes can often see well without glasses,
but it takes work. They must use their focusing mechanisms
just to make distant objects clear. Nearer objects require even
more effort to keep in focus, so for long spells at the computer,
those with uncorrected hyperopia often tire and experience
eyestrain.*

**Astigmatism.** *Astigmatic eyes have irregularly curved lenses
that create a blur no matter what the distance. Usually
associated with myopia or hyperopia, astigmatism correction
is built into their solutions. One study revealed that even small
amounts of uncorrected astigmatism can lead to reduced
performance at the computer.*

**Presbyopia.** *Presbyopia is the natural loss of focusing ability
that comes with age. See **The Aging Eye**, page 16. Bifocals,
often prescribed for presbyopia, sometimes lead to neckaches
at the computer. Solutions include glasses customized to your
monitor's distance and angle.*

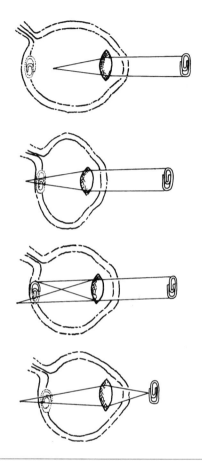

- Generally, computer users stare at the screen for long periods,
  placing stress on the muscles that focus and direct the eye.

- Computer users often make the same eye movements repeatedly, fatiguing their eye muscles.

- The more light the eye has to work with, the more distance
  behind and in front of an object the eye keeps in focus. When
  this distance (the depth of field) is short, the eye has to work
  harder. Many computer screens aren't very bright, decreasing
  the depth of field that the eyes can maintain in focus. This is
  especially true of monitors that display light letters on a dark
  background.

## Eye Warnings

If you experience any of these symptoms, you should seek an immediate eye examination.

- A profound change in vision

- Eye discomfort for any prolonged period

- Wandering eyes or double vision

- Finding you cover one eye when you read

This is not a comprehensive list.

- Computer users often work in dry environments, and tend not to blink often, which decreases the lubricating layer of tears on the eye.

### How You Can Tell You Might Need Glasses

The American Optometric Association (AOA) suggests that the following symptoms of visual stress indicate you might need your eyesight corrected.

- Frequent headaches

- Tired or burning eyes

- Blurred vision

- Frequent accidents

- Difficulty parking

- Difficulty reading the newspaper or other small print

- Poor sports performance

- Decreased interest in tasks requiring close work

## Examine Your Examiner

The AOA suggests you have an eye examination before you begin computer work and follow-up exams at yearly intervals. That may be going a bit far, but if you have any kind of existing eye condition, it's worth considering an exam before problems arise. Finding an eye-care professional who can solve the problems associated with computers can sometimes be vexing and challenging. Here are some tips, plus some eye-related warning signs of more serious health problems.

Increasing numbers of eye-care professionals understand the special factors involved in computer-related eye issues. But some are not as up to date in the field as others. A good eye-care professional is conscientious about analyzing visual function at near-work distances, and should work with you to design occupational glasses if they are called for.

When you make an appointment, be sure to mention whether you think you may have a computer-related eye problem. If you are asked to bring measurements of the distances and angles from your eyes to your screen, keyboard, and documents to the examination, then the examiner probably has the experience you want. If you aren't asked for these measurements on the phone or during the office visit, you should consider another examiner.

## Finding the Right Correction

Glasses and contact lenses may pose special problems at the computer; many commonly prescribed bifocals, trifocals, and contact lenses aren't designed for use with computers. Wearing them may cause symptoms that seem unrelated to vision. The solution may be a dedicated pair of spectacles or contact lenses customized for your computing environment.

**Computer glasses.** Computer glasses are usually designed for the distance and angle at which you view your monitor. Although the expense of buying an additional pair of glasses can be annoying, for many the resulting decrease in eyestrain is well worth it. About 40 percent of those who see optometrists about a computer-related eye problem receive lenses customized to computer work.

**Bifocals.** Bifocals prescribed for presbyopia commonly contain a lower lens set to focus at 16 inches or 40 cm that extends down from the elevation of the lower eyelid. This works well for reading material on a desk or in your hands, but necessitates cocking the head back and moving it forward to clearly see a computer screen—a "chicken dance" that can result in neck and back strain. To correct this, examiners may prescribe bifocals in which the top lens corrects for objects at monitor distance (with the bottom lens set for closer work). Another solution might be computer glasses. Some people may find relief by lowering their monitors. Another problem of standard bifocals is that their viewing area is too small to keep the entire screen in focus. Larger bifocals may be prescribed to overcome this problem.

> ■ ■ ■
> **Glasses and contact lenses can be customized for computer work.**
> ■ ■ ■

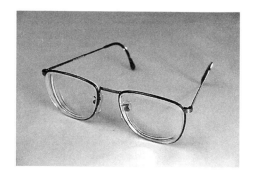

# The Aging Eye

As the eye ages, its ability to change focus diminishes and finally disappears, a condition known as presbyopia. The aging eye requires more light to see accurately, while at the same time it becomes more sensitive to glare. Tear production decreases.

## Presbyopia

A normal human eye focuses over a range of distances from very close to very far away by using the ciliary muscles to change the curvature of the lens in the eye. As we get older, the lens hardens and we lose that ability. We are less able to adjust our focus, which makes it difficult for us to see nearby objects, including computer screens. This natural loss of near vision is called presbyopia. Initially, presbyopia is treated with bifocals. But as the condition progresses, the area we can't focus on becomes deeper, and another lens is often added (going from bifocals to trifocals), yielding three distances of accurate focusing.

## Light Sensitivity

Our pupil becomes less reactive to light the older we get. It becomes smaller, allowing less light to enter the eye, and, as a result, we need more light to see well. Additionally, there is a tendency for the lens of the eye to yellow, and for cataracts (clouding of the eye's lens) to develop. These cataracts, although small, can scatter light—making bright lights or reflections a much more visually incapacitating problem in the older eye than the younger.

## Tear Production Reduction

Tear production decreases as one ages, especially in women. The eye needs the lubrication of tears to function properly. Computer use already strains the maintenance of a proper tear layer, so age-induced tear reduction is particularly onerous at the computer screen. Dry eyes feel scratchy, and become red and irritated. See **Eyestrain**.

**Trifocals.** Trifocals may have their center lens focused at the correct distance for computer work, because that lens is often customized to a wearer's specific need. However, the position or small size of that lens may cause a trifocal wearer to perform an annoying chicken dance. Computer glasses or special bifocals may offer a less stressful alternative.

**Progressive addition lenses.** Progressive addition lenses contain variable-power lenses: the top part focuses on objects far away, while the lower parts focus on progressively closer objects. As you look down the lens, the focusing power of the lens changes gradually, so that you have a more normal change from looking at the distance to looking up close. Many wearers find typical progressive addition lenses taxing for long periods at the monitor because of the inherent distortion in the peripheral field. However, some newer models have a wider area of clear vision, so are less stressful.

**Contact lenses.** Normal contact lenses are designed to focus at 20 feet and therefore may not be adequate for nearer distances, especially at the lower illumination levels encountered in many video displays. At the computer, contact lens wearers are particularly susceptible to dry eyes, and the accompanying irritation. Sometimes computer glasses are prescribed to be worn over contacts. Also, bifocal contacts can be a satisfactory solution—but not for everyone.

■ ■ ■

**Get the visual correction that's best for your working conditions.**

■ ■ ■

## Resources

See **Where Else to Turn** for a complete list of companies, products, associations, and other helpful resources.

*20/20: A Total Guide to Improving Your Vision and Preventing Eye Disease*, Mitchell H. Friedlaender and Stef Donvev (Emmaus, Pennsylvania: Rodale Press, 1991).

**American Academy of Ophthalmology**, PO Box 7424, San Francisco, CA 94120-7424. (415) 561-8500.

**American Optometric Association**, 243 North Lindbergh Blvd., St. Louis, MO 63141. (314) 991-4100.

# 4 Headaches

**Pain You Can Do Without**

*Headaches come in many varieties.*

■ ■ ■

**The office is a minefield of headache sources.**

■ ■ ■

**Related chapters:**

- Stress
- The Perfect Workstation
- Lighting
- Monitors

Headache producers are common in the office environment. Headache triggers include deadlines, heavy work loads, repetitive and monotonous tasks, air quality (fumes and perfumes), and glaring lights. It's a rare workstation that's not stocked with pain relievers, but dependence on pain relievers can backfire, causing more headaches. A variety of measures can bring relief.

## Headache Types

Headaches appear in different sizes, shapes, and varieties; their exact causes are debated, with much still unknown. Many specialists view the causes of most types of headaches on a spectrum, linked by the complex interrelating functions of the brain and the nervous and musculoskeletal systems of the neck and head. But most common headaches are lumped into two general categories.

### Tension
Long hours at the computer can be a prime source of tension headaches—the most prevalent of all headaches suffered. Tension is a catch-all phrase used to describe a variety of headaches linked to a tensing, or contracting, of the head and neck muscles, causing pain. These muscle contractions are related to many factors, including stress, anxiety, fatigue, and body strains and pains. Pain can be severe or mild, last for minutes or hours, and affect the whole head, or specific areas. Tension headaches can be chronic or occasional.

### Migraine
For some computer users, glare and flickering fluorescent lights may bring on migraine headaches. Migraines are linked to disturbances in the vascular system (blood vessels) serving the head and

# Where It Hurts

*Pain pathways of common headaches.*

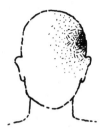 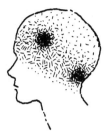 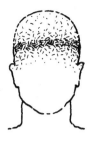 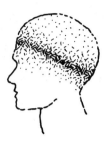

**Migraine.** *Pain is usually most severe on one side of the head, but can be generalized. It often affects the entire body, primarily causing stomach problems and visual disturbances.*

**Tension.** *A variety of headaches fall into this category, from occasional stress aches to chronic pain. Aching is often accompanied by a sensation of pressure. Tension headaches can affect all or any part of the head.*

---

brain, and seem to be hereditary. Migraines are often triggered by external stimuli: light, noises, certain foods, stress, pain, the menstrual cycle, and even smells, like paint fumes. In other cases, the cause is unclear.

Usually attacking one side of the head, migraine headaches can be excruciatingly painful, tend to recur, and may affect the whole body, causing stomach and vision problems. Sufferers may experience nausea, vomiting, lack of appetite, blurred vision, or acute sensitivity to light. Migraines can also be mild. They last from a few minutes to days. Migraines are often preceded by visual disturbances, such as focusing problems or seeing stars or "auras."

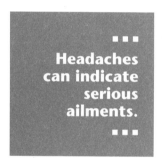

**Headaches can indicate serious ailments.**

## Less Common

Found within the arenas of both tension and migraine headaches, or in between, are several less common sources of head pain. Ice cream, coughing, depression, sinus problems, and even sex can cause headaches. Cluster headaches—severe episodes of pain (typically around or behind on eye) recurring daily for several weeks or months—are believed to be akin to migraines. Mostly affecting men, clusters hit, then months or years can pass before another attack. Headaches can also be symptomatic of an underlying illness or condition, such as a tumor, infection, or disease.

## Instant Migraines

Some specialists report that sitting in front of a video screen for a short period of time—five to 30 minutes—can trigger migraines in *a small number* of people. It's believed that certain characteristics of light emitted by the monitor can play a role in eliciting a migraine. Should this occur, see your doctor. Antiglare screens, dark glasses, and adjusting screen color and brightness may help. If these bring no relief, computer work may simply not be advised.

## What to Do

Pay attention to the intensity and frequency of headaches. Don't be a martyr: headaches can indicate serious ailments. If they bother you, see a doctor. A combination of preventive tactics and medication can almost always help ease your pain.

### Prevention

Some migraine sufferers can determine what prompts an episode and then try to avoid the triggers. With chronic tension headaches, experimentation may be necessary to find what best dents the annoying pattern. Try the following.

**Limit stress.** Maintaining a relaxed and comfortable work environment is one of the most effective ways of preventing tension headaches. See **Stress**.

**Reduce muscle strains and pulls.** Work at a comfortable workstation that adequately supports the upper body, neck, and shoulders. Get a telephone headset; a standard telephone handset causes strain when crooked against your neck. See **The Perfect Workstation**.

**Optimize your view of the screen.** Make sure the monitor is directly in front of you at an appropriate distance and height. Eliminate reflections in the monitor. Consider an antiglare screen (but realize they are not a panacea—some can reduce clarity and increase eyestrain). Experiment with screen brightness and contrast. See **Lighting** and **Monitors**.

**Focus on fresh air.** If you smell something funny, such as paint fumes or solvents, report it; some fumes can cause headaches and worse health problems. If a co-worker has donned a new perfume around the same time you started getting headaches, politely suggest a switch—either in perfume brand or workstation location. See **Office Air**.

**Watch what you eat.** Certain foods trigger headaches in some people. Pay attention to intake of sulfides, present in many red wines; monosodium glutamate (MSG), found in Chinese and many prepared foods; and nitrites, often found in meats, and in aged and processed cheeses.

## Treatment

Some remedies may help all headaches; others are specific to one headache type.

■ Migraine sufferers should be under the care of a doctor; most find relief with prescription medications.

■ For an occasional tension headache, analgesic pain relievers—aspirin, ibuprofen, or acetaminophen—should do the trick. Avoid chronic use. If headaches persist; see a doctor. See **Medications**.

■ Either cold or hot compresses can ease a variety of headaches. But migraine sufferers beware: the application of heat can often worsen migraines.

■ Relaxation techniques—such as biofeedback, meditation, and relaxation exercises—may help.

## Resources

See **Where Else to Turn** for a complete list of companies, products, associations, and other helpful resources.

**National Headache Foundation,** 5252 North Western Avenue, Chicago, Illinois 60625. (312) 878-7715. Provides information on request.

Most cities and major hospitals have headache clinics; consult your Yellow Pages under **Hospitals**.

## Coffee's Clutch

Caffeine affects the opening and closing of blood vessels, and both excessive caffeine and caffeine withdrawal can cause headaches. Watch excessive intake of caffeine-containing substances, like coffee or many soft drinks. If you've decided to swear off lattés after making them a lifestyle (the so-called "Seattle syndrome") you may want to reduce your intake gradually. Traditionally, many common pain medications have contained caffeine, and recent research suggests that caffeine heightens the pain-relieving effect of its accompanying analgesic. Ironically, many people with chronic tension headaches pop caffeine-containing pain relievers every day to relieve headaches, but are actually bringing headaches on.

# 5 Lighting

## Balancing Illumination and the Monitor

Lighting designers know that different tasks require different amounts of light; the more intense and exacting the procedure, the more light is necessary to accomplish it satisfactorily. Computer users, although operating in a visually demanding environment, are burdened by screens that only emit a limited intensity of light. And because the eyes naturally adjust themselves to the brightest light in their range of vision, if other lights are brighter than the monitor, the eyes strain to focus on the screen. Light sources in the work area must often be moderated and controlled to ensure they don't overpower the screen, create bright spots in the operator's field of vision, or produce annoying reflections.

Traditionally, offices have been brightly lit for working with paper, which is not necessarily a good environment for working with computers. In a study of New York City offices, only 10 percent had good visual environments for using computers. Most offices have some or all of these lighting woes.

■ Glare on walls and surfaces

■ Reflections on screen

■ Excessively bright light from windows and skylights

■ Excessively bright light from fluorescents and incandescents

■ Bright areas in the field of vision

Luckily, a few simple steps usually suffice to make a big difference, so that office lights work with—rather than against—the computer screen.

## Real World Lighting Solutions

Good lighting gives people control over light sources of the proper illumination and design.

# Balancing Act Between the Light Sources

*These light producers must be properly adjusted or modified to yield the correct balance of lighting (the luminance ratio). The golden rule is that luminances of objects within your field of vision that are near your screen should be less than three times brighter than the screen itself. Objects that are more distant should be less than 10 times brighter than the screen.*

**Reflections in the screen.** *Light sources behind and above the operator may need to be louvered, repositioned, or otherwise modified to kill reflections. Dark letters on a light background mask reflections. Glare shields or hoods may be necessary. See* **Monitors**.

**Exterior.** *Exterior luminance can be extremely bright, so reduce it with blinds, partitions, or tinted windows. You may need to modify workstation placement to reduce bright spots in the field of vision.*

**Interior.** *Modify interior luminance to conform to the correct luminance ratio. Neutral or dark paint can decrease the luminance or reflectivity of walls.*

**Light from screen.** *The maximum working brightness of your screen is the starting point for your light balancing act. Dark background screens require lower overall lighting to achieve the desired balance.*

**Light on your copy.** *Working-material brightness ratios should conform to the luminance ratio. If you use a task light, ensure it is neither too bright nor spills any direct, bright light into your field of vision.*

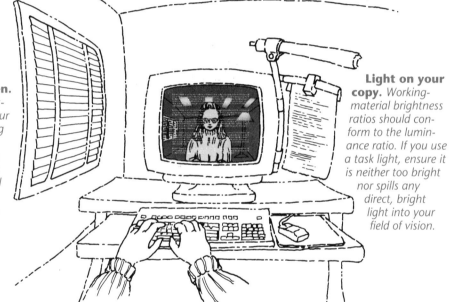

## Power to the People
The perfect lighting design is elastic and accessible—it must adjust to the changing conditions of the office environment and the different needs of its inhabitants.

**Make the lighting adjustable.** The light surrounding a workstation often changes. Office lights go on and off, and daylight—even attenuated by blinds—is sufficiently powerful to

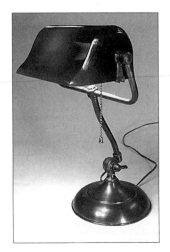

create significant shifts in the overall ambient light levels during the course of the day. Lighting design must be adjustable enough to adapt to these changing conditions.

**Give people control.** Not only should the lighting adjust, but its adjustment should be in the hands of the people who need it. Lighting requirements vary between individuals depending on age, workstation geography, computer screen, and job type. In order to achieve the optimum visual environment, computer users should be consulted as to their particular requirements, given access to lighting adjustment, and trained in proper adjustment.

## Lighting Standards

There are a mind-boggling variety of office lighting statistics and standards, often using exotic measurement systems, and they're often misinterpreted when it comes to practical application. Yet those standards can be reduced to a few practical principles.

**Similar luminances.** Luminance represents the brightness of an object, which is different from illuminance (how much light falls on an object). A dark object that's brightly illuminated has a low luminance. The fundamental principal for good lighting is that you should have similar luminances in the field of view of the computer user. In other words, when you look at your computer screen there should be no "hot spots" of light noticeable behind or around the screen. Furthermore, objects you look at for your task (the screen, reading material, keyboard, and so on) should be of similar brightness.

**Maintain the luminance ratio.** The Illuminating Engineering Society (IES) suggests that the luminance of what you are concentrating on (like your computer screen) and its immediate surroundings (like your copy) should vary by no more than a factor of three. The luminance of more remote objects (like a window beyond your screen) should not be more than a factor of 10 times brighter than your screen. You can get a good idea if you are in the luminance ballpark by using a camera with an good internal light meter. See *How to Measure the Luminance Ratio*, page 26.

**Keep ambient light at the right level.** The current American National Standards Institute (ANSI) lighting standard for work-places with VDTs prescribes ambient (overall) illumination in the range of 200–500 lux (18–46 footcandles), which may be too low for many offices; the advent of white-background computer screens allows a higher ambient illumination level than the older, "black hole," dark-background screens. Note that this is an illumination standard; in most situations you can arrive at a satisfactory ambient light level by using the luminance ratio discussed above. This usually requires modifying already existing light sources.

As a general rule, keep any bright light sources as far away from the field of vision as possible. Use blinds, drapes, or tinted glass to reduce the outside light to an acceptable level. Because daylight varies in intensity, adjustable lighting is especially helpful. Inside, you probably need to cut down the intensity of fluorescent banks, which can be accomplished simply by removing some of the tubes. Some fixtures can be retrofitted with parabolic louvers— directing the light downward and eliminating the reflections they can cause.

### Task Lighting: Use with Caution

Task lights can help reduce reflections and provide ample light in a small area, perfect for lighting documents at the computer, especially when the ambient light level is low. However, task illumination is misused more than it is properly used, more often than not producing too much light for the proper luminance ratio. Also, task lights are often incorrectly positioned or louvered—throwing bright light straight into the eyes of the computer user.

### Control Bright Lights and Surfaces

Bright areas in the field of vision often go unnoticed— but can cause visual stress. Sit at your workstation and then shield your eyes. If it feels better, you have a problem. Any distracting bright lights or surfaces with a luminance greater than 10 times that of your screen should be dealt with.

## Fluorescents Flicker?

Flicker, a rapid oscillation of light, can produce eyestrain when it is evident in the monitor (see **Monitors**). By investigating the flickering of fluorescent lights, Dr. Arnold Wilkins at the Medical Research Council Applied Psychology Unit in Cambridge has suggested that unperceived flicker may cause eyestrain. Although most people don't perceive flicker above 65 hertz (Hz), the eye still reacts to it at rates up to 125–160 Hz. Dr. Wilkins examined the eye problems reported by workers operating under fluorescents—both with normal flicker and with a flicker rate much higher than the eye responds to. There was significantly more eyestrain in the normal flicker environment. At least one lighting expert suggests that people who may be especially sensitive to flicker should mix in a significant amount of non-flickering light (sunlight or old-fashioned incandescents) with any fluorescents.

# How to Measure the Luminance Ratio

*Any good SLR camera with a built-in light meter can be used to derive a workable approximation of the luminance ratios around your workstation. You set the film and shutter speed, and the camera indicates luminance levels with the f-stops it suggests to use. Here's how to do it.*

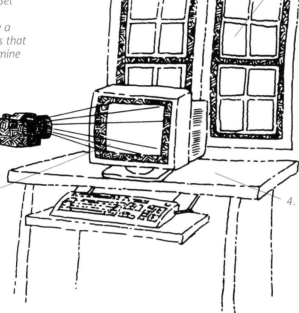

1. *Set the ASA to 400. Set the speed to ¹/₆₀ of a second. This will give a good range of f-stops that you will use to determine the ratio.*

2. *Make the largest white area (or light area, if your screen isn't white) you can on your screen. Position the camera so the white area fills the frame. Write down the indicated f-stop.*

3. *Look for the brightest object in your field of vision. Fill the frame with the light source (moving toward or zooming into it as necessary) and write down the f-stop. This reading should be within 3¹/₂ stops of the reading in step two.*

4. *Put a piece of white paper where you usually keep documents, fill the frame, and write down the f-stop. This reading should be within 1¹/₂ f-stops of the reading in step two.*

**Bright lights.** Control lights with baffles, louvers, or blinds. Turn them off or put a plant in front of them. Fluorescent lights can be difficult to control, so consider turning them off and bringing in an incandescent or halogen floor lamp that bounces light off the ceiling or walls to produce a soft, indirect illumination. Many people claim that these continuous spectrum lights are easier on the eyes than fluorescents. Consider repositioning your workstation. You can easily notice potentially annoying reflections by looking for them in your screen before you turn it on. See **Monitors**.

**Surfaces.** Office walls may be too bright if their color is too light or their glossiness produces shiny reflections. Painting white walls a pale gray, green, brown, or orange can cut reflective glare in half. Flat-finish wall paint reflects less than a gloss or semigloss. Fabric-treated walls cut luminance and glare.

## Resources

See **Where Else to Turn** for a complete list of companies, products, associations, and other helpful resources.

**Illuminating Engineering Society of North America**, 120 Wall Street, 17th floor, New York, NY 10005. (212) 248-5000. Publishes *Lighting for Offices Containing Computer Visual Display Terminals* (1989) for $35 plus $3 shipping.

# 6 Monitors

## Making It Easy on the Eyes

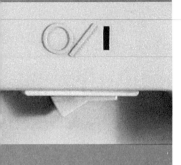

*A precise image helps you avoid eyestrain.*

■ ■ ■
**Simple measures can reduce glare.**
■ ■ ■

**Related chapters:**

- Lighting
- Eyestrain
- Glasses and Contact Lenses

Your monitor should display a precise image, free from distractions which might cause eyestrain. Achieving this image requires a capable and adequately adjusted monitor, with its content legibly displayed. This chapter investigates those monitor characteristics that affect how you see. Because the monitor is merely one creature in the office ecosystem, you might want to also check out the chapters on its close relations—**Lighting, Eyestrain,** and **Glasses and Contact Lenses**.

## Choosing the Best Screen

Choosing a monitor can be daunting. If you were able to compare a wide selection of monitors placed side by side, you could appraise their relative image quality. Because such a comparison is generally not feasible, even in the largest computer stores, many popular computer magazines (*PC, PC World, MacUser,* and *Macworld,* in particular) publish periodic in-depth comparisons of monitors that contain objective testing results and subjective analyses that can help you make an intelligent choice. In a few cases, the technical specifications published by the monitor manufacturers can be helpful. Here's a rundown on what you need to know to choose a less stressful screen.

### Focus

The eye continually refocuses on a blurry image in a vain attempt to make it clear. Over time this results in eyestrain. When the eye evaluates screen focus, it takes into account sharpness (how tight the electron beam is and how closely packed the screen's phosphors are), convergence (how well the three electron beams in a color monitor coincide in space), and how much glare the screen image is throwing back. Sharpness and convergence can be measured electronically, and most magazine reviews combine those results with subjective evaluations of focus.

# A Visually Satisfying Screen

*Several factors combine to deliver a pleasing view from your monitor. Monitors need to be cleaned frequently to display the most accurate picture. Periodic degaussing may also be necessary.*

**Focus.** *Picture appears crisp and sharp; not out of focus.*

**Surface treatment.** *Choose the best for your lighting environment.*

**Brightness.** *Sufficient brightness for your lighting environment.*

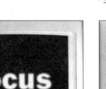

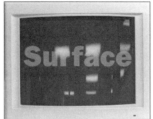

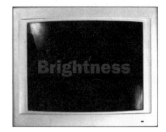

**Display.** *Characters or graphics are easily legible.*

**Flicker.** *Screen is free from flicker.*

**Contrast.** *Higher contrast enhances legibility.*

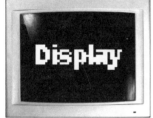

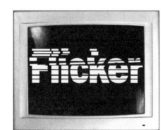

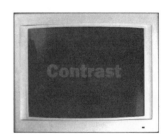

## Brightness

More than any other property, brightness can vary dramatically from one monitor to another; you might need a brighter screen if the ambient light in your office is high and cannot easily be controlled (see **Lighting**). Higher brightness also masks glare and yields higher contrast—both favorable characteristics. Ultimately, there is a trade-off between brightness and sharpness: some monitors can be adjusted so brightly that their image becomes fuzzy; but because screen phosphors fade in time, in a few years this adjustment may yield a perfect picture. Other monitors have restricted brightness, keeping a sharp, albeit darker, image. Magazine reviews are the easiest way to get stats on a monitor's relative brightness.

# Liquid Crystal Displays

Liquid crystal displays (LCDs), used on most laptop computers, represent a number of technological compromises: as a rule they are small, slow, lack sufficient contrast, can't be seen at too wide an angle, and are unusually susceptible to glare from ambient lighting conditions. All of those problems can be visually distressing. And yet some can deliver surprisingly crisp and pleasing images. There are a few different types of LCDs, which vary in price and visual quality. Before you buy one, try it out—preferably in the conditions you expect to work under—to ensure that it doesn't become a site of sore eyes.

**Passive matrix without backlight.** This LCD must be used in a location with ambient lighting, because reflected light serves to illuminate the light areas on the screen. This handicap leads to very low contrast and the ability to display black and white only (or more accurately, dark gray and light gray only)—both distinct disadvantages. On the plus side, these LCDs are relatively inexpensive, lightweight, and use the least power.

**Passive matrix with backlight.** The backlight allows for much greater contrast and the possible use of grays. But up until recently, these screens were only available with slow refresh rates, so the cursor often submarined (disppeared) as it moved. Some new passive-matrix screens feature "dual-scanning," which delivers twice the refresh rate of standard passive screens, producing a significantly sharper image. Color passive-matrix displays exist, but lack good saturation. Weight and power consumption increase along with the visual quality.

**Active matrix.** Active matrix LCDs are the best of the lot, providing more contrast, wider viewing angle, and a faster response time. The color models give adequate color rendition. Active matrix displays cost a bundle, but they're coming down steadily.

## Flicker

Flicker is a pulsing or strobing of the screen image due to a low refresh rate (the time it takes the electronic beam to "repaint" the picture). Flicker rates that are barely perceptible to the eye nevertheless cause the eye to continuously readjust, causing fatigue and headaches. Manufacturers usually publish the refresh rate under the specification titled something like "Vertical Refresh Rate" measured in cycles per second, known as hertz (Hz). A vertical refresh rate above 70 Hz produces a flicker-free picture for most viewers (in larger or brighter screens, flicker is more apparent). However, about 10 percent of the population is particularly sensitive to flicker; if you are one of those people, you might need to view the screen to ensure that you can tolerate it. Both magazine reviews and manufacturer's specifications contain refresh-rate values.

Check the scanning pattern of the monitor and display card; "interlaced" scanning methods scan every other line, so they need two passes to create a complete picture; "noninterlaced" techniques scan every line, every time. Most modern display systems are non-interlaced because they produce less flicker, but some of them switch to interlaced mode for higher resolutions.

## Surface

Screens vary in their curvature; those that are flatter give fewer reflection problems. Less expensive monitors often have more curve to the surface. Most screens are treated in some manner to reduce their reflective properties. However, all surface treatments represent compromises.

**Silica coated or etched.** These two processes yield screens which diffuse light that hits them from the front. However, these treatments cause the picture to lose contrast and become somewhat fuzzy. Generally, this still yields a image sufficiently precise for most viewers; manufacturers (and buyers) like these treatments because they are relatively inexpensive.

**Thin-layer coatings.** Two types of thin-layer coatings are used on monitors, one better than the other. Optical coatings like those used on camera lenses significantly reduce glare while allowing for maximum light transmission. Unfortunately, dirt—especially oily dirt such as fingerprints—show iridescence like an FBI agent's dream evidence, prompting frequent cleaning. Optical coatings cost a lot, so most manufacturers avoid them. They excel in situations where glare is a severe problem.

The other thin-layer coating is called "quarter wave," and it works by creating two reflections that partially cancel each other out—reducing reflections less successfully than optical coatings.

Whether or not your screen has an antireflective coating, you might want to consider a glare filter, discussed below.

### Adjustability

Many monitors include adjustable stands that tilt and swivel to accommodate your particular workstation. Avoid excessively redirecting the monitor to reduce reflections and glare. The controls that you use the most—power switch, brightness, contrast, and sizing—should be easily accessible. If you want to maintain a precise display by adjusting your monitor, you should look for one that also has accessible convergence, focus, and pin-cushion controls. However, these adjustments are not for everyone—both experience and testing software are helpful.

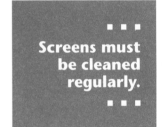

**Screens must be cleaned regularly.**

## Making Your Screen Work for You

The best monitor in the world will give you eyestrain if it is positioned incorrectly or if what you display on it is difficult to view.

### Position

Position your monitor more than 18 inches (45 cm) from your eyes. Monitor placement should allow a downward gaze angle to all parts of the screen. Traditional advice placed the top of the screen at eye height, but some experts now suggest that lower may be better. According to Denny Ankrum, Human Factors Analyst for Nova Office Furniture, the top of the monitor should be tipped back at much the same angle you use when reading a book. That improves vision and may reduce neck and backaches.

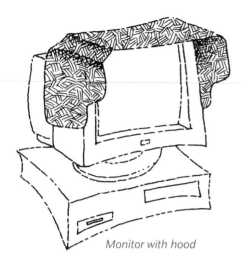

*Monitor with hood*

But, Ankrum warns, glare problems must be addressed at the same time or the benefits will be negated (See *Glare and Reflection Reduction*, page 32). If you are worried about electromagnetic radiation from the monitor, you may want to keep it at a greater distance (an arm's length) but be aware that you may have to increase the size of type and other display elements (or even get a larger monitor) to compensate. See **Radiation**.

### Colors and Contrast

Use colors intelligently. Some people get a color monitor and go Hollywood, making their type green, the background red, and their boldface blue. Although the judicious use of color can make images clearer, it's hard to concentrate on many different colors simultaneously; adjacent areas of red and blue are particularly difficult to focus on. And different monitors have varying success in displaying different colors. So use common sense. When displaying text, you want as great a contrast between the letters and their background as possible.

### Type Height

Small type is hard to see. Type that is too large slows down your reading, and makes you scroll around more within a document. What's just right? It depends on you and the resolution of your video setup. Do what feels best for you. If you find yourself leaning into the screen to see, it may be that your type is too small (or you need vision correction; see **Glasses and Contact Lenses**). Some monitors may not have sufficient resolution to display smaller font sizes adequately, so make sure the font you choose is legible. The matrix of dots making up a character should be at least $7 \times 9$. If you find it difficult to scan a line of type, then the type may be too large.

### Glare and Reflection Reduction

If slightly repositioning your monitor or adjusting lights doesn't reduce glare or reflection, you might try a good cleaning or a hood. If neither works, consider a glare shield (see *Glare Filters*, page 34).

**Cleaning.** Cleaning your screen is the easiest way to substantially increase your monitor's performance;

a clean screen is brighter and produces more con-trast—both qualities that reduce the effects of glare and reflections. How often you need to clean your screen depends on the screen's surface coating type and the amount of dust it attracts (color monitors generally attract more than monochrome). But clean your screen regularly—certainly before the dust becomes noticeable.

Most screens can be cleaned with a nonscratching towel (available from many computer stores and catalogs) moistened with glass cleaner (or a weak solution of soap and water), followed by a damp towel rinse and a wipe clean. But always follow the manufacturer's cleaning instructions, when available. Be careful: Some coatings and plastic screens scratch easily. Attempting to clean these could damage them and render them worse then before.

**Hoods.** Hoods can offer a simple and inexpensive solution to reflections in the screen. Although available from manufacturers, they can be construc-ted out of cardboard and tape with a minimum of skill. Black cardboard with a matte finish is best.

### Degaussing

Occasionally, a magnetic field may build up around your monitor, degrading the image. Usually, the problem is signaled by a shift in color on one of the sides or corners, especially with a move toward pink or blue. Some monitors have a built-in degaussing (demagnetizing) feature, triggered by a push but-ton, but most screens automatically degauss when you turn them off and then on again. If this doesn't work, your problem may be due to external mag-netic fields. See *Screen Gone Psychedelic?*, page 35.

### Adjustments

If you are bothered by screen flicker, try checking your monitor and graphics board specifications. You may find you can increase your vertical refresh rate to a higher, less noticeable, value. However, don't arbitrarily jack the rate up to its maximum; by doing so, you may significantly decrease the sharpness of the image.

As screens age, image quality degrades and brightness becomes less uniform. Without your

## Black on White? White on Black?

Most experts agree that black char-acters on a white background are easier to see than vice versa: people are used to viewing printed text in that form, and a large white field reduces the effect of screen reflec-tions. But your monitor must be up to the job.

Producing a bright white back-ground taxes many color monitors because all three electron guns are firing at their maximum intensity. Some monitors actually dim slightly when large areas of white are displayed because of protection circuits built into the tube. Also, due to a slow refresh rate, flicker is more noticeable when large bright areas are displayed. Try correcting either of these difficulties by changing the background to a light green or blue, making sure you maintain a high contrast between the background and the principal objects (like text).

If you work with a dark back-ground on your display, be sure to minimize reflections in the screen through lighting control and monitor positioning—and, yes, some people even resort to wearing a dark shirt so they won't see themselves reflected in the screen.

## Glare Filter Seal of Acceptance

The American Optometric Association has recently begun a program that evaluates and approves glare screens. Look for an AOA Seal of Acceptance as one indicator of a glare filter's optical and construction quality and effectiveness in reducing glare (see **Resources**).

being aware of it, your screen's alignment may have drifted, and may be causing eye fatigue. So your screen may need to be adjusted periodically—how often depends on the screen and how picky you are. If you purchase a used monitor, check it out immediately.

If you suspect your monitor is not at its optimum, you can take it into the shop to get adjusted for about $50 or $100. Or adjust it yourself—a task that's made easier with the appropriate software (see *Resources*, page 35).

A final warning: Don't try to adjust internal controls unless you know what you are doing; the voltages can be lethal, even after the monitor has been off for a while.

## Glare Filters

Filters can magically change the appearance of your screen display—sometimes for the worse, and sometimes for the better. The resulting image depends on the filter's type, its quality, and your lighting and monitor conditions.

Glare filters are made either of a hard glass or plastic, or of a loosely woven mesh. Most increase your screen's contrast by reducing the reflected glare more than the emitted light. Reflected light must pass through the filter twice, while light emitted from the monitor passes through only once. Some filters are electrically conductive and designed to be grounded, reducing both the electrostatic field and the electrical component of the electromagnetic field produced by monitors, and also reducing the monitor's attraction of dust. See **Radiation**.

It is best to try a filter to make sure it is effective for your work area, so find one with a money-back guarantee.

**Hard filters.** Most hard filters carry antireflective coatings like those used on monitors (see *Surface*, page 30), to both reduce glare and overcome their introduction of two additional potentially reflective surfaces. Additionally, hard filters function by increasing contrast through a tint or polarization application. Polarization can be a particularly effective glare-reducer for certain kinds of glare.

Because the attachment of a hard filter often leaves a gap between filter and screen, they can trap dust, and some create more reflection problems than they solve. Generally, the closer they are mounted to the screen (some adhere to it) the better. Optical purity is a necessity, and can be lacking, particularly in the plastic models.

**Mesh filters.** Mesh filters act as a dark, matte scrim, allowing light to pass out from the monitor while absorbing light hitting it at a different angle. They are particularly effective when there is a bright light reflecting directly off the screen. On the down side, mesh filters partially obscure the screen image, can reflect light coming from certain angles, and can create moiré patterns.

## Resources

See **Where Else to Turn** for a complete list of companies, products, associations, and other helpful resources.

**DisplayMate**, Sonera Technologies, P.O. Box 565, Rumson, NJ 07760. (800) 932-6323. The most advanced diagnostic testing software for monitors. $149.

**American Optometric Association**, 243 North Lindbergh Blvd., St. Louis, MO 63141. (314) 991-4100. Certifies quality glare filters.

## Screen Gone Psychedelic?

Has your monitor developed colored blotches that shift when you rotate it? Does your electric pencil sharpener make your screen dance the hula? A magnetic source (other monitors, laser printers, and stereo speakers are common culprits) may be affecting your screen. Sometimes degaussing will make things right again. Otherwise, identify and move the offending article. If that doesn't work, you might check out the JitterBox from NoRad (see **Where Else to Turn**). Other common problems include a bad power supply causing flicker (get the power supply fixed), or power lines causing a shimmering or pulsing in some screens (try repositioning, or switch to a model less sensitive to outside interference). A flickering or swimming screen may warn you of a strong electromagnetic field you may wish to avoid (see **Radiation**).

# Radiation

## Smoking or Saccharin?

You're sitting outside a large conference room filled with scientists, industry experts, and government officials, all debating whether or not radiation emitted by power lines, computer monitors, and the wiring and appliances in homes and offices is dangerous. Three people walk out, and you ask, "Should I be worried about it?" They answer in order: "Absolutely; it causes cancer!"; "We don't know; we need to study it more"; and "No; there are no convincing studies that show how it can hurt you."

What do you do?

First, realize that this is how science works. One scientific model does not replace another overnight. Sometimes a usurping theory is shown to be false, and sometimes it becomes the new accepted theory—but not without debate. That debate is influenced by the persuasiveness and reproducibility of data, and—in the case of biological hazards—the toxicity of the material in question.

Until recently, the electromagnetic radiation emitted by monitors (which includes the type of radiation emitted by power lines) was thought to be benign. Over the last 15 years, a small number of studies have challenged that assumption, suggesting that chances of developing leukemia and other cancers, and the odds of miscarriage, may increase with prolonged exposure to certain narrow bands of electromagnetic radiation.

Most people find it difficult to weigh the risks from electromagnetic radiation because the subject is complex, the radiation invisible, and reports seem contradictory and often are sensationalized by the press. Further confounding judgment is the fact that some of the emissions from monitors are similar to those found all around us in our "electrical civilization." Although you cannot predict how the scientific debate will be resolved, you can arm yourself with the facts and be your own judge on what you should do.

# The Electromagnetic Spectrum

*We live in a sea of electromagnetic energy. Naturally occurring electromagnetic energy—sunlight, for example—fills only very discrete sections of the electromagnetic spectrum. The rest of the spectrum is filled by electromagnetic radiation (EMR) produced by civilization, such as television signals, radar, and X-rays.*

*The wide range of frequencies that make up the electromagnetic spectrum are measured in cycles per second, or Hertz (Hz). They can also be indicated in higher frequencies by wavelength, noted below in micrometers (μm, one millionth of a meter) and nanometers (nm, one billionth of a meter). Higher frequencies carry more energy, and those frequencies above the ultraviolet carry enough energy to break chemical bonds and cause biological change. Called ionizing radiation, this high-frequency radiation has been considered hazardous for some time.*

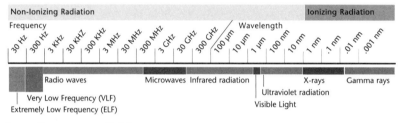

## Low-Frequency Fields

*Controversy now surrounds the safety of low-frequency electromagnetic fields (EMFs)—principally those generated by power lines (60 Hz in North America), but also those emitted by monitors. Power line EMFs are in an extremely low frequency portion of the electromagnetic spectrum—hence they have been dubbed ELF (extremely low frequency) fields. Computer equipment generates ELF fields, and some fields in the very low-frequency (VLF) area of the spectrum.*

*Since the dangers of these low-frequency fields have not been proved, it is not known if ELF fields are more dangerous than VLF fields, though some of the studies suggest ELF is more hazardous. Some scientists have speculated that biological damage occurs at specific frequency "windows" or may be exacerbated by the more exotic sawtooth or square-wave patterns generated by monitors.*

---

# The Electromagnetic Field Debate

Scientists' and experts' opinions about the toxicity of low-frequency electromagnetic fields vary widely.

## Point/Counterpoint

Those who have concluded that VLF and ELF fields are hazardous cite as evidence the results from a number of studies. On the opposite side are experts who have concluded that the evidence

# Magnetic and Electric Fields

One of the most perplexing aspects of EMFs is that they can be either of two types of field—electric or magnetic. These two types of fields produced by monitors are blocked by different materials; for example, a grounded conductive screen will block the electric field but allow the magnetic filed to pass, whereas magnetic fields can be absorbed by some unusual metal alloys. The results of one clinical study suggest that the monitor's magnetic fields pose a greater biological risk than the electric fields.

is insufficient to prove a danger exists. Many of these detractors reason that even if a danger were proven, it will turn out to be slight and does not warrant the attention and money spent for investigation and remedy; many more lives could be saved by concentrating on more pressing health problems. Other scientists say that they need more evidence before they can decide on the dangers of VLF and ELF fields.

**Epidemiological studies.** Four major studies, in Denver, Los Angeles, and Sweden, suggested childhood leukemia was two to four times higher near power transmission lines or in homes with wiring rated for heavy electrical loads.

Other epidemiological studies (the first from the former Soviet Union, followed by others in the United States and one recently in Canada) showed a surprising variety of adverse health effects (including a wide variety of cancers) in people who have occupational exposure to power lines (like electric utility workers).

Detractors point out a number of problems with these results. Other power-line studies have not demonstrated any correlation to leukemia in children. A follow-up to the Los Angeles study eliminated many environmental variables unrelated to electrical power which were included in the original, and showed there was no correlation between the leukemia incidence and the strength of the power-line fields. Plus, occupational power-line studies have come to inconsistent conclusions: one indicates that brain tumors result from exposure, while another indicates leukemia.

Detractors also point out that even if power-line exposure were shown to be dangerous, computer monitors may not pose the same risks. They also question the validity of using epidemiological studies to demonstrate a relationship, because such studies only show a correlation between two factors; they can't demonstrate a cause-and-effect relationship. For example, you can't conclude that because Haitians have a high incidence of AIDS, being born in Haiti causes AIDS. Epidemiological studies that demonstrate low dangers (like 2 to 3 times normal levels) are statistically less valid than they would be if they showed that the danger were higher.

**Cellular and animal studies.** Studies have shown that cancerous cells in culture demonstrate accelerated growth under power-line-generated magnetic fields. Detractors point out that fields generated by monitors and power lines are sufficiently different that potential biological hazards of power lines can't be attributed to monitors. In other studies, chicken and mice embryos developed abnormally when exposed to low-frequency magnetic fields. Detractors note that waveforms used in the chicken-embryo study were not the same waveforms as those emitted by VDTs, making the results inapplicable to monitors. Finally, detractors argue that you have to make a big jump to transfer the results of animal studies like these to humans.

### Draw Your Own Conclusions

One argument voiced by some who have concluded ELFs are safe is that there has been no cause-and-effect relationship shown; no study has demonstrated how this radiation causes cancers or miscarriage. But others point out that proving a clear cause and effect often isn't always necessary for a substance to be regarded as toxic, as long as the other evidence is convincing.

For example, asbestos (a clearly toxic substance) was considered dangerous before it was known exactly how it killed people. In the United States, society expects its government to regulate toxic substances, and generally that regulation has been good. But there are exceptions, like cigarettes, which are clearly toxic but are still legal.

Saccharin, on the other hand, was regulated mostly based on rat studies that were ultimately shown to be inapplicable to human beings. (Rats, unlike humans, appear to have an enzyme that changes saccharin into a carcinogen; plus, the rats in these studies were given tremendous amounts of saccharin.) So far, the United States government has not found the evidence for ELF and VLF dangers compelling enough to warrant regulation.

It's worth noting here that when a possible hazard is carried prominently in the media, people view it as being more dangerous. When saccharin was linked

## Monitor X-Rays?

Monitors, like televisions, produce X-rays, a form of ionizing radiation that can harm living tissue. But not to worry: these X-rays are contained *inside the tube,* and so pose no health threat. Some early television sets did emit X-rays, but manufacturers modified their design in two ways; these same X-ray reduction methods are used in monitor manufacturing today. First, manufacturers include circuitry that limits operating voltages, capping the strength of the X-rays produced. And second, to contain these X-rays, lead salts are mixed into the glass of the tubes, completely blocking any harmful X-ray transmission. Several studies have detected no X-ray emissions from large samples of typical office monitors. So devices that claim to block dangerous X-rays emitted by your monitor just aren't needed—save your money.

## Field Reduction Retrofit

If you have an older monitor that produces strong magnetic fields, two companies make products that may help. NoRad Corporation's ELF ProTech flexible bands attach to the sides of your monitor and absorb the magnetic fields (to some extent). Safe Technologies can retrofit a compensating coil around the yoke of your monitor that it claims will reduce the emissions to MPRII guideline levels. This device must be installed at the factory. See *Resources*, page 43.

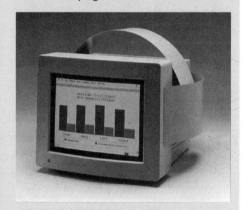

*NoRad's ELF ProTech*

to cancer, the media reported on it widely, and so the public perceived it as a more dangerous substance than most scientists did.

Major monitor manufacturers say they want this issue settled; many now shield their monitors and fund studies on monitor radiation. No one knows how the radiation debate will finally turn out—whether EMFs from monitors or from electrical wiring and powerlines will be proved to be a health hazard. For now, you can do nothing, knowing that you live in an electrical society and that the evidence of toxicity is not compelling to many experts. Or, you can take some easy precautions to minimize your exposure to monitor EMF.

## Reasonable Precautions

If you are worried about EMFs from monitors, it's simple to do a few things to reduce your exposure. But be aware that becoming psychologically stressed by this issue can possibly harm you more than the radiation. See **Stress**.

**Use a monitor that conforms to MPRII or TCO guidelines.** If you're shopping for a monitor, consider one that meets the Swedish National Board of Testing's MPRII guidelines (the abbreviation comes from the board's Swedish initials) or the more stringent guidelines of TCO, the Swedish white-collar labor union. Although neither guidelines' field levels are proven as safe, they are much lower than those emitted by most older monitors.

**Stay an arm's length away from your screen.** If you don't have a lower emissions monitor (like one that's MPRII-compliant), staying an arm's length (about 30 inches or 75 cm) from the screen drops the EMFs to the background levels found in most offices. If this new distance makes your monitor harder to view, you may need to increase the size of objects on your screen (such as text). Stay four feet or about 1.2 meters away from the back and the sides of monitors, since fields can be stronger there. And be aware that walls and partitions don't block these fields.

# EMFs at the Computer

*Various components in your computer generate electromagnetic fields at various wavelengths and with various wave forms. In modern computer equipment, these fields may be so well shielded as to be below environmental background levels.*

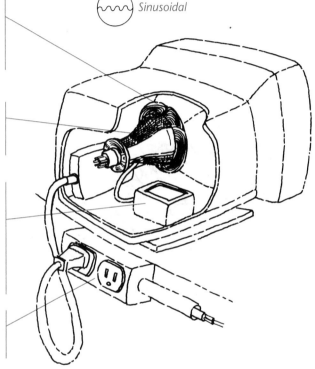

Sawtooth

Square

Sinusoidal

**Flyback transformer and horizontal deflection coil.** *The flyback transformer creates high-voltage sawtooth waveforms from 15–45 kHz. This current passes through the horizontal deflection coils, forcing the electron beam to sweep horizontally across the face of the tube.*

**Vertical deflection coil.** *The vertical deflection coil steps the scanning beam down the face of the tube. It primarily generates a square wave form, typically from 50–90 Hz.*

**Power transformer.** *The power transformers in your monitor and computer both generate sinusoidal 60 Hz fields. The computer's power transformer is well shielded to ensure that its radiation does not interfere with nearby components. Modern monitors may match the low emission levels of the power transformer.*

**Electrical power.** *Electrical power from wiring, lights, and equipment radiates 60 Hz fields throughout most offices and homes.*

---

**Turn your monitor off when not in use.** It's easy to reduce most of the EMF exposure (and save electricity) by just turning your monitor off when it's not in use. According to the Environmental Protection Agency (EPA), 80 percent of the time a monitor is operating, it isn't being viewed. Many new computers and monitors comply with the EPA's Energy Star program, automatically powering down or going to a lower-power state when not in use.

**Consider special precautions if you are pregnant.** Some experts suggest you limit your time on the computer if you are pregnant, or trying to become pregnant. See **Pregnancy.**

## Consultants

It may give you some peace of mind to know the strength of the electromagnetic fields where you live or work. However, there is no accepted way to interpret the health effects of any measurements. If you are still interested, consultants are available who will measure electromagnetic field strength. Look for them in the phone book under "Environmental Services" or "Engineering." Be forewarned that people without adequate expertise also advertise themselves as consultants. The chances are that electrical engineers will know what they are doing.

If you are concerned about the emissions peculiar to monitors (in addition to power-line EMFs) you should make sure your consultant can measure them. A typical rate for such service is around $75 an hour. Residences take about two hours to measure; businesses are often charged at a higher rate.

## Staying on Top of the Field

If you are concerned about EMFs, you might want to reduce your exposure to other sources in the environment. Keeping adequately informed as the issue unfolds should help determine what's best for you.

### Consider Other EMF Sources

We live in an electrical society; we are exposed to EMFs in almost all parts of it, often from hidden sources. If you are worried about EMFs, it may not make sense to reduce exposure to your monitor while there are much more potent EMF emitters in your environment. However, it's questionable how much you can practically reduce your exposure, and what this reduction might mean to your health.

**Be aware of the worst offenders.** In the home, older electric blankets may pose a serious risk as they are close to the body for long periods of time. Many electric shavers, can openers, and power tools generate strong ELF fields, and are generally operated near your body (though for shorter periods). In the office, desk lamps and some laser printers and photocopiers generate significant ELF fields.

**Measure your exposure.** Many power companies will measure ELF fields free of charge. You can buy a testing meter and measure the ELF fields yourself, but you might want help (see *Consultants*, at left). Be advised that while meters in the $100 range can accurately measure the magnetic fields of power-lines, they can be fooled by the higher frequencies and exotic waveforms produced by a monitor, and yield inaccurate measurements. And even if you have a good measurement, how you interpret it becomes a significant issue, because no level is proven as safe—or dangerous. However, after taking high readings from transmission lines, power companies have sometimes been known to reduce the fields by a process known as reverse phasing.

## Inform Yourself

As more studies on ELF fields are completed, the issue should become clearer. If you're concerned, it may be worth your while to stay current on the topic.

**Read.** *VDT NEWS* provides the most comprehensive reporting on this subject (see *Resources*, below). The better computer magazines report on this issue well (*Macworld* has taken a leading position in covering the subject); some major newspapers may be as precise, others may not. Look for conclusions by government agencies, such as OSHA and NIOSH in the US, and the Workers' Compensation Boards in Canada, but keep in mind that they may be influenced by politics.

**Don't be misled.** The complexity of the subject matter and the lack of scientific study lends itself to confusion. Read material diligently—especially from those that have an ax to grind or a buck to make.

## Resources

See **Where Else to Turn** for a complete list of companies, products, associations, and other helpful resources.

***VDT NEWS***, PO Box 1799, Grand Central Station, New York NY. (212) 517-2803. *VDT NEWS*, a newsletter covering the industry, has long been the peerless source of monitor EMF information. Year's subscription (6 issues) for $127. A list of all the magnetic field meters currently available in the United States is also available for $1 (include a self-addressed stamped envelope as well).

**NoRad Corporation**, 1160 E. Sandhill Ave., Carson, CA 90746. (310) 395-0800.

**Safety First Organization**, 1400 Opus Place Suite 960, Downers Grove, IL 60515. (800) 432-4513.

> ■ ■ ■
> We live in an electrical society.
> ■ ■ ■

# 8 Pregnancy

## The Computer's Uncertain Effects

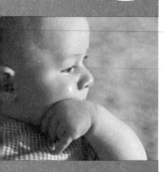

*Assessing the risk to the mother and the developing fetus.*

■ ■ ■

**A few precautions can reduce dangers to the developing baby.**

■ ■ ■

Can working at a computer damage you as a pregnant woman, or your developing baby? Maybe, but probably not—especially if you take a few simple precautions. Psychological stress—whether computer-related or not—can endanger your developing child, and should be minimized. The jury is still out on the dangers of electromagnetic radiation, so how you react to it becomes a personal decision. Your own health while pregnant may be adversely affected from sitting too long. Plus, pregnancy increases the chances of getting carpal tunnel syndrome and De Quervain's disease, conditions that are both also related to computer use.

While this chapter is focused on personal choices that women must make, its information should also be of use to men, to help them better understand the issues facing women in the workplace. Managers and supervisors should especially take note.

## Danger on the Desktop?

Smoking, diet, chemicals, medications, garden work, exercise—it seems like nearly everything can affect the health of a developing baby. So it wasn't surprising when about 15 years ago research began indicating that computer work might be added to the list. First, mysterious groups of miscarriages were reported, then a major epidemiological study linked miscarriage to computer use.

- In 1980, reports of offices where women experienced increased rates of miscarriage began to appear in the press. Whether these "cluster miscarriages" were caused by electromagnetic radiation, constrained sitting, stress, or some other factor associated with computer work wasn't determined, and still isn't known. Subsequent research led many experts to discount most of the clusters as statistically normal: if you look for a condition within a large population, a few groups with high rates of the

44

condition appear due to chance alone. Or, it may been due to faulty methodology. However, these reports raised the issue of computer safety in the minds of the both the public and many scientists.

■ In 1988, a study of 1,583 pregnant women by the Kaiser Permanente health maintenance organization found "a significantly elevated risk of miscarriage for working women who reported using VDTs for more than 20 hours per week during the first trimester of pregnancy." Much of the press treated the Kaiser study as a bombshell, even though a number of prior studies elsewhere had shown no statistically relevant association between miscarriage and computer work.

Many of the press reports suggested the miscarriages were due to electromagnetic radiation, yet the Kaiser researchers clearly stated that they were not postulating a biological cause for the results—although they discussed stress, electromagnetic radiation, poor ergonomic conditions, and recall bias (of the women in the study) as possibilities for the outcome. The researchers suggested that more studies were necessary to clarify the issues.

After the Kaiser study, a number of studies were proposed and funded. Another retrospective study (some of the information comes from the subjects recalling how much time they spent in front of computers—a technique vulnerable to scientific criticism) should be released soon from Kaiser Permanente. A "prospective" study (the researchers take the measurements as they follow the subjects) at Mt. Sinai Hospital in New York should be out in the next few years.

Other recent studies have shown no correlation between computer work and miscarriage. For example, a large Danish epidemiological study released in late 1992 found no correlation between miscarriage and computer use. A significant study by the National Institute of Occupational Safety and Health (NIOSH) released in 1990 found no correlation between miscarriage and very low frequency (VLF) electromagnetic fields generated by monitors. But a seemingly contradictory result came from a Finnish study, published in 1992, which found a correlation between exposure to a high level of ELF fields and increased rates of miscarriage. These studies are discussed on pages 47 and 48.

**Questions remain, yet risks (if they exist at all) appear minimal.**

## Informed Opinion

For now, most experts view the evidence for computer-related miscarriage as being far from conclusive. Those who feel a mother's computer use is safe for a developing fetus argue that if it were otherwise, some of the studies with negative outcomes would have been positive. Other experts feel enough studies show a correlation to warrant care and further study.

If a problem does exist, scientists have yet to determine which of the many aspects of the computer environment might be causing it. Until more studies yield results, seek your doctor's advice, follow the well-known suggestions that have been proved to produce a healthy child, stay informed of the issues, and take sensible precautions if they ease your mind and help reduce your stress level.

## Baby's Health

Psychological stress, a factor that's often associated with computerized offices, can be the cause of negative pregnancy outcomes, but how much stress causes damage varies considerably between women and situations. The effect of electromagnetic fields on the developing fetus is far more controversial. Some studies suggest a relationship between miscarriage and electromagnetic fields; others don't. If electromagnetic fields turn out to be harmful, they are probably a minor factor compared to other day-to-day health issues, and a few simple steps can bring your exposure down to the level of the everyday environment.

■ ■ ■
**Reduce your psychological stress load during pregnancy**
■ ■ ■

### Stress

Psychological stress can result in adverse pregnancy outcomes, but exactly how you and your doctor apply this knowledge takes some care. As a rule, you want to reduce your psychological stress load during pregnancy, but people have different reactions to stressful situations. Because many women need or want to work through their pregnancies, and because stress can be beneficial, you and your doctor need to determine the best level for you. (See **Stress**.)

An interesting study demonstrated the capricious nature of stress and pregnancy: 1,283 pregnant medical residents who worked 70-hour weeks were tracked to see if their high-pressure jobs affected their pregnancies. Their pregnancies were statistically normal.

### Electromagnetic Fields

Research has not proven a link between electromagnetic fields and miscarriage or birth defects. Although a few animal studies showed fetal damage resulting from magnetic fields, and a new epidemiological study suggested a link between extremely low frequency (ELF) fields and miscarriage, other results have been negative. A recent British review of VDT pregnancy studies found no support for risk. More research must take place before the issue can be proven one way or another. (See **Radiation**.)

**Animal studies.** A few animal studies have demonstrated a correlation between magnetic fields and abnormal fetal development. Although some scientists feel these experiments suggest the need for more research, no one suggests they prove a link between computers and miscarriage.

■ Between 1982 and 1988, first in Spain and then elsewhere, experiments that exposed chick embryos to pulsed magnetic fields showed inhibition of normal growth and development. These experiments were confirmed, but have been discounted by some scientists because the magnetic fields were dissimilar to those associated with computers.

■ A 1986 Swedish study of pregnant mice exposed to low-frequency, sawtooth waves similar to those made by computers resulted in significantly increased fetal malformation and death.

**Recent human studies.** Two recent human studies investigating the relationship between computers and miscarriage have shown differing results.

■ In 1990, a NIOSH study concluded that "the use of VDTs and exposure to the accompanying electromagnetic fields were not associated with an increased risk of spontaneous abortions." This study compared pregnancy outcomes between telephone operators who worked with computer monitors and those who worked with LED screens. The study reportedly suffered from political intervention, reducing its scope (sections concerning fertility and stress were removed). Also, the study considered only very low frequency (VLF) fields; ELF exposure for the two groups was identical, and went untested. Many scientists argue that ELF exposure is the more damaging of the two types of radiation, and therefore denigrate the overall value of this study.

■ A Finnish study published in the *American Journal of Epidemiology* in late 1992 concluded that "exposure to a high level of extremely-low-frequency magnetic fields of video-display terminals in early pregnancy may be related to spontaneous abortion [miscarriage]. However, the possible risk apparently applies only to a small proportion of the video-display terminal users."
  The study asked women to recall the amount of time they spent at a computer during a previous 10-year period and evaluated this information using equipment EMF measurements derived from previous studies. No correlation between miscarriage and VLF exposure was shown. However, those women in the ELF high-exposure group showed 2.8 times greater miscarriage rates when compared to a combined group of VDT users with

low ELF exposure and women who didn't use VDTs at all. Although this rate is statistically significant, it is small.

The authors of the study called for further studies using precise measurements of exposure, and studies of females in other electrical environments in order to see if this correlation between miscarriage and ELF exposure could be duplicated.

See **Radiation** for more background on ELF and VLF issues, including the MPRII standard for monitors.

**What to do.** Some experts say pregnant women should reduce their exposure to electromagnetic fields; others say the evidence is not sufficiently conclusive to warrant concern. If you have had trouble conceiving or carrying a child to term, you may want to exercise additional caution regarding factors that may cause miscarriage. Many women who have decided to reduce their exposure to electromagnetic fields have negotiated with their employers for reduced time at the computer, for transfer to another job while pregnant, or for purchase of a low-emission monitor. (For other reduction methods, see **Radiation**.)

Don't use a lead apron, which does nothing to block these fields, but poses a risk to your fetus by pressing on it.

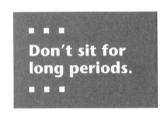

**■ ■ ■**
**Don't sit for long periods.**
**■ ■ ■**

## Mother's Health

Not only the developing baby, but the mother might also be subject to health risks at the computer. Those who are expecting may want to be careful about sitting for long periods, and be aware that computer work could worsen some consequences of pregnancy—notably carpal tunnel syndrome (CTS).

### Sitting

Pregnancy causes fluid retention. That fact coupled with the tendency of pregnant women to be less active means that when they sit, they often experience a fluid build-up in their legs and feet. This discomfort can be minimized if you remember not to sit for long periods; get up and stretch and move. If the condition continues to bother you, consider a 20-minute rest in the afternoon lying on your left side, which can promote circulation and reduce the buildup of fluid. Off the job, swim, walk, or partake of other moderate exercise to promote good circulation.

As a rule, sitting on the job seems to be good for your developing child. Those women who stand in fixed positions while they work (for example, hairdressers and dentists) have about twice as many premature births as those who sit on the job. (Work that involves standing but moving, like waitressing, gives even fewer premature births than sitting). However, women sitting in the constrained postures associated with computer work have not been specifically studied, so there may be more information for computer users in the future.

### Carpal Tunnel Syndrome and De Quervain's Disease

Up to 35 percent of pregnant women—whether they work on the computer or have never seen one—experience carpal tunnel syndrome or De Quervain's disease during or immediately after pregnancy. (See **Shoulders to Hands** for a description of these conditions.) These maladies may occur due to hormonal changes that lead to an the increase in fluid retention and swelling.

Normally, pregnancy-related CTS disappears immediately after the birth, and De Quervain's often subsides sometime after birth. Because of their transitory nature, both conditions may be treated with splints; if this is not effective, doctors may prescribe steroid injections (after the baby is weaned) or surgery. Prudence suggests that you seek a second opinion before resorting to surgery. (See **Getting Medical Help**.)

Does computer work accelerate or aggravate CTS and De Quervain's disease? Doctors don't know for sure, but it has been suggested that computer work may be a factor. If you are pregnant or plan to get pregnant, tell your doctor about your work at the keyboard (she'll want to know anyway). If you believe you may have either condition, be sure to inform your doctor, and don't forget to remind her about the time you spend at the computer.

## Resources

See **Where Else to Turn** for a complete list of other resources, including organizations providing information and consulting.

**VDT NEWS**, PO Box 1799, Grand Central Station, New York, NY. (212) 517-2803.

**9to5, National Association of Working Women**. (414) 274-0925. Organization focuses on several issues affecting office workers, including reproductive risks.

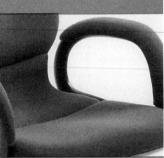

# 9 The Chair

## Sitting on the Job

Sitting is a compromise. You sit to reduce the strain on many of your muscles, allowing them a chance to rest and recuperate. But, simultaneously, other muscles work to keep you sitting. And if you don't move, these muscles cause fatigue and pain as lactic acid, the by-product of muscle activity, builds up in your tissues.

Humans are not designed to sit. Even if your posture is perfect, the pressure on the lumbar disks (the doughnut-shaped cartilage between the vertebrae in your spine) increases by 30 percent when you are seated. Chair-related injuries range from minor aches to permanent disk damage (see **Back and Neck Pain**).

Originally, seats and backs were two flat rocks set at right angles, and for many years "proper" seated posture maintained this ramrod straight body position with elbows and knees set at 90 degree angles. Studies by NASA in zero gravity demonstrated that a relaxed body configured itself somewhere between sitting and lying down, and now experts can't agree on the best seated posture, and exactly how reduced physical stress (in other words, comfort) relates to injury levels.

The most recent thinking suggests that how your body feels should guide you, so the emphasis is on comfort; to be comfortable you need a chair that can accommodate a range of postures throughout the workday. With this, there is a growing acceptance of a seat pan that's able to tilt forward. But not all chairs—even those that appear to be on the forefront of design—are based on modern ergonomic principles. You must find the chair that fits you and your job, and adjust it and use it properly, to prevent injury at your computer.

*The relaxed body in zero g.*

# The Lumbar Curve

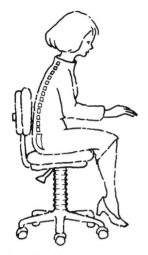
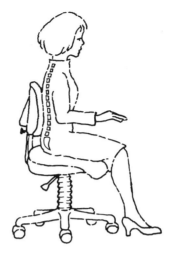

*An unhealthy lumbar curve*          *A healthy lumbar curve*

# Warning Signs

Various aspects of chair design and adjustment can cause trouble. Areas of discomfort can be interrelated; but most stem from an incorrect seated posture. Watch out for these warning signs that suggest your chair is working against you.

### Lower Back Pain

Lower back pain can develop from a poor seating posture (slouching) when the lower lumbar region's natural inward curve flattens or reverses. A chair can cause you to slouch in a number of ways.

- The chair might be too low or too high, causing you to bend forward to do your work.

- The chair surface that supports the lumbar spine region may not be sufficiently curved (or adequately adjusted) to hold the spine in the proper position.

- Your chair may be too far from your monitor, causing you to lean forward to see.

- Your feet may not be supported, causing you to sit on the front edge of the seat so you don't use the back for support.

- In rare cases, the seat pan may be tilted too far backward, so that your knees are drawn up toward your stomach, causing the lumbar curve to flatten.

> ■ ■ ■
> **Perhaps the best tip for safe sitting is to stand up occasionally.**
> ■ ■ ■

**51**

# The Perfect Chair

*A good chair is comfortable, adjustable, and adaptable: it maximizes support and minimizes stress while encouraging you to assume different positions without "hot spots"—areas where the chair presses on parts of the body, causing discomfort. The best design accommodates your workstation, tasks, body, and work intensity. If you use a computer intensively, you need an ergonomically designed chair; if you are up and down constantly, you might not require as sophisticated (and expensive) a model.*

**The right size.** *Chairs are like shoes: you need one in "your size," and some just fit better than others. People who are heavy, short, tall, or thin are all likely to need different chairs. You need to test a chair out, either at your workstation or in a showroom where you can mimic your work conditions, and then adjust your chair correctly to find the best fit.*

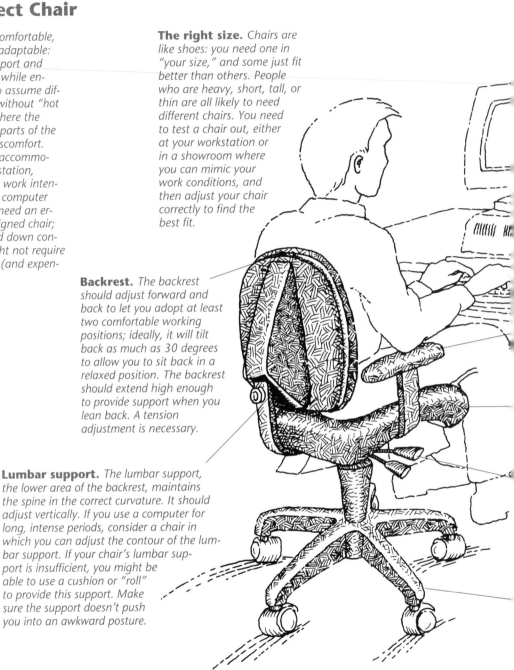

**Backrest.** *The backrest should adjust forward and back to let you adopt at least two comfortable working positions; ideally, it will tilt back as much as 30 degrees to allow you to sit back in a relaxed position. The backrest should extend high enough to provide support when you lean back. A tension adjustment is necessary.*

**Lumbar support.** *The lumbar support, the lower area of the backrest, maintains the spine in the correct curvature. It should adjust vertically. If you use a computer for long, intense periods, consider a chair in which you can adjust the contour of the lumbar support. If your chair's lumbar support is insufficient, you might be able to use a cushion or "roll" to provide this support. Make sure the support doesn't push you into an awkward posture.*

**Height.** *The height adjusts so you can hang your arms straight down from your shoulders with your elbows bent 90 degrees to allow you to comfortably place your fingers on your keyboard with your wrists in a neutral position (but don't hold this classic posture for too long). For many people, this means your legs have about an inch of clearance under your workstation or desk, but this can vary depending on your torso and arm length. Your feet should be flat on the floor or a footrest. People will more likely adjust the height of chairs that have pneumatic height adjustments.*

**Armrests.** *Armrests need to be padded and close enough to lean on without straining. They should adjust vertically and not hit or scrape on your workstation because it prevents you from getting close enough to your keyboard and monitor. Experts are undecided as to whether or not your forearms should contact the armrests while you are typing.*

**Pan.** *The seat pan is padded and contoured for support while allowing movement, and is never so long as to touch the leg below your knee. The front slopes down and the surface provides enough friction to keep you from sliding—but not so much friction to prevent you from easily shifting position. The pan can be adjusted to tilt forward to give you a range of comfortable working positions. If you lean forward for a significant part of your work day, a forward tilting pan becomes more important.*

**Adjustable while sitting.** *The chair should be adjustable while you're sitting in it. This makes it easy for you to change your position.*

**Foundation.** *Five legs reduce the chance of accidentally tipping, and castors increase movement. The chair should feel solid. Most people prefer a chair that swivels, but you may not need that feature.*

# Kneeling Chairs

Many ergonomists feel that the flaws of kneeling chairs far outweigh the advantage of the chair's forward-tilting seat. Kneeling chairs put stress on the knees, tire the back, and when their occupants try to stand up, these chairs can spill them onto the floor. If used at all, kneeling chairs should be reserved for short breaks from a chair with a sounder design. If the forward-tilted pelvis position appeals to you, an ergonomically designed chair might give you all the forward adjustment you need.

## Sleeping Feet

Legs or feet falling asleep could be due to a badly designed or adjusted seat pan that presses into the underside of the thigh. Or sleeping feet might come from a chair that's too high when you don't have adequate foot support.

## Upper Back- and Neckaches

Upper back- and neckaches can result from slouching, improper upper back support, not leaning against the back of the chair, or from a chair that is pivoted away from your monitor.

## Tailache

Aching in the tailbone results from pressure on the end of your spine (the coccyx). It can result from a slouched posture which tilts the pelvis bones—which usually support the seated body—out of the way, so the body's weight rests on the end of the spine. A poorly contoured seat that presses into your tailbone can also lead to the condition.

## Wrist- and Armache

Wrist- and armache can be due to a chair that's too high or too low, causing you to hold your hands and wrists in stressful positions.

## Use Your Chair Correctly

The best chair design in the world won't overcome improper use. To minimize chair-induced injury, sit smart. Good sitting means moving. Adjust your chair to accommodate your body. Don't be afraid to kick back, but beware of putting tension on your body by using the keyboard while assuming "relaxed" positions.

**Move.** Throughout the day, shift your position frequently to relieve muscle tension. Take proper breaks away from the chair. See **Schedules.**

**Adjust.** Adjust your chair to provide comfort; your body should feel relaxed, with nothing pressing into it. If you don't know how to adjust your chair, find out. It's in management's best interest for you to be seated properly.

**Relax.** Sometimes your body may be telling you to put your feet up. Go ahead. Although this may seem to be an "unprofessional" posture, stretching out for short periods reduces pressure on your discs and allows fatigued muscles to relax and recuperate.

## Buying the Right Chair

Your chair may be with you longer than any other piece of office equipment, so it pays to find one that's right for you. Well-made chairs can appear expensive—until you consider the value of its occupant's work, especially in the light of medical and disability costs. A well-made chair should also last for 20 years (so it should see you through at least seven computers at today's turnover rates). The budget-minded can sniff out savings of 50 percent at showroom sample sales. Chairs that carry the tag "ergonomic" may or may not be; there is no organization that certifies this quality. Get a long tryout period for your purchase and return it if not satisfied.

## Resources

See **Where Else to Turn** for a complete list of companies, products, associations, and other helpful resources.

***Hard Facts about Soft Machines: The Ergonomics of Seating***, Rani Leuder and Kageyu Noro (Washington, DC: Taylor and Francis, 1993).

***American National Standard for Human Factors Engineering of Visual Display Terminal Workstations***, Human Factors and Ergonomics Society (HFES), PO Box 1369, Santa Monica, CA 90406. (310) 394-1811. Includes specifications of safe chair design. A new standard should be released in 1995.

## Take the Posture Test

Are you unsure whether you are sitting correctly? Good posture is usually evident to the eye, so have a co-worker check out your posture at your workstation. Work alone at home? Pull your chair over to a full-length mirror and check yourself out.

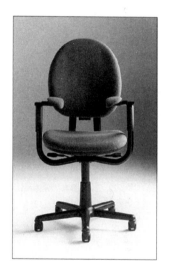

*A good chair offers a solid foundation, several easy-to-reach adjustments, and lumbar and arm support.*

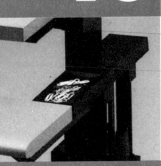

# 10 The Desk

## Putting It All on the Table

*Your desk should function like a cockpit.*

■ ■ ■

**Height depends on task.**

■ ■ ■

**Related chapters:**

- The Chair
- The Perfect Workstation
- Beck and Neck Pain
- Shoulder to Hands

It is not unusual to see an office where the chairs, management, and training follow ergonomic standards, but where rows of desks are contrived from simple tables not designed to facilitate the diverse tasks at hand. Or, perhaps each workstation's surface has been installed at the same height, even though their occupants are of drastically different sizes.

Too often the desk represents the lost component of furniture purchasing, even though desks—especially their heights—can be critical to preventing cumulative trauma disorders (CTDs), neck- and backaches, headaches, and other problems endemic to computer users.

## What to Do

A desk should function like a cockpit—perfectly adapted to you and your work. The key is the height of your keyboard, but you also need to consider legroom, workspace, and clutter.

**Different jobs require different designs.** Jobs have different space requirements—a graphic artist may require much more flat space than a data-entry clerk. Analyze your work, perhaps by not- ing the different time and space requirements for each major task, then make sure you have enough workspace for each element of your job. Don't forget to reserve space for storage and telephone. Desks need to provide ample room for your legs and feet, so you can shift your position without hitting anything.

**Different bodies require different heights.** You need to adjust your workstation so it fits you. Adjust the surface on which your keyboard sits so that your wrists are in a neutral position. If

# The Dangerous Desk

*Improper desk design or setup can cause discomfort and predispose you to injury.*

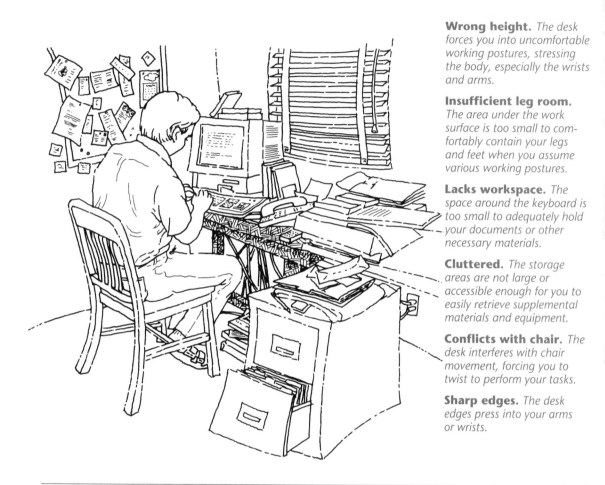

**Wrong height.** *The desk forces you into uncomfortable working postures, stressing the body, especially the wrists and arms.*

**Insufficient leg room.** *The area under the work surface is too small to comfortably contain your legs and feet when you assume various working postures.*

**Lacks workspace.** *The space around the keyboard is too small to adequately hold your documents or other necessary materials.*

**Cluttered.** *The storage areas are not large or accessible enough for you to easily retrieve supplemental materials and equipment.*

**Conflicts with chair.** *The desk interferes with chair movement, forcing you to twist to perform your tasks.*

**Sharp edges.** *The desk edges press into your arms or wrists.*

you are forced to raise your chair to attain this position, then use a footrest. Consider adjustable-height surfaces to accommodate different tasks or various postures you may adopt throughout the day. Make sure your chair adjusts to the various work surface heights and nestles close enough to give you comfortable working positions and space to fidget.

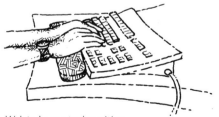

*Wrists in neutral position.*

## Stand Up, Sit Down Solution

Intensive computer users may want to consider a workstation which adjusts to a standing configuration. When Pacific Bell acquired a few standing workstations for their directory assistance operators, they proved so popular that, to handle demand, operators were limited to 30-minute shifts.

**Arrange your work materials.** A place for everything and everything in its place. Your primary work area should contain necessary materials well within easy reach. Store frequently needed materials close by, within an arm's length if possible. Don't place something so it requires you to stretch too far—better to get up and walk. See if you can move the main box of your computer out of your way, perhaps onto the floor (but make sure you aren't blocking its ventilation and causing it to overheat).

## Keyboard Holders

Keyboard holders can provide an easy solution for desks that are the wrong height—if you have the right keyboard holder and use it correctly. Simple pullout trays may be sufficient, but you should ensure that they actually provide the keyboard height you need. Keyboard supports on cantilevered arms offer more adjustment; the best can be positioned above the desk surface as well as below, and don't bounce. If you use a mouse, make sure your keyboard holder provides ample room to use it. Reaching past the keyboard holder to use a mouse on the desk can create problems. Keyboard holders are not ideal with all jobs—for example, some people find there is no place for writing materials when using a keyboard holder.

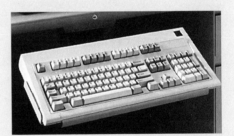

# Keyboards and Mice

## Pitfalls and Hands-On Solutions

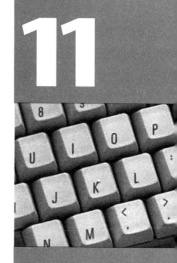

Keyboard design has been held hostage by history. Legend has it that the standard QWERTY layout was adopted on early mechanical typewriters because of the need to separate the striking bars of letters most often typed sequentially, thus reducing the chances of the bars fouling.

Although this explanation is probably apocryphal, the QWERTY layout may be one of the contributors to cumulative trauma disorders (CTDs) in computer users. To what extent and exactly how layout and other factors like keyboard geometry relate to injury is virtually unknown.

Manufacturers have been slow to develop alternatives because of lack of adequate scientific guidance and limited demand. Businesses hesitate to buy any design that would take more than a few days to master. And the fear of product-liability lawsuits plays a role—manufacturers don't want to admit that what they make may be dangerous (although now some manufacturers, including Microsoft, are putting warning labels on their keyboards).

However, the input device revolution has begun: a number of new devices have appeared recently. But before you go out and buy one of these alternatives, arm yourself with as much knowledge as possible; remember that it isn't just the equipment that makes a difference, but how you use it. And be forewarned that many new designs will appear and disappear before a new standard emerges.

## Keyboard Essentials

Most well-made standard keyboards offer these features.

**Detachability.** You must be able to position a keyboard so it's comfortable. An extra-long keyboard cord may be needed.

**Thin profile.** A thin profile keeps the keys lower, making it more likely you can adjust your chair and desk correctly to keep your

*It's unknown just how much keyboard and mouse design contributes to cumulative trauma disorder.*

■ ■ ■

**Alternatives range from simple layout changes to voice input.**

■ ■ ■

## Related chapters:

- Shoulders to Hands
- The Desk
- The Perfect Workstation

# Good Typing Technique

Even the most well-designed and configured equipment may not protect you from injury if you don't use good typing technique. It's easy to fall into bad habits, so try to be aware of how you position yourself when you type.

**Float hands and wrists.** Use the larger muscles of your arms to position your hands to help reduce stress on the smaller muscles in your fingers. Use wrist rests and chair arms for support when you are *not* typing.

**Type lightly.** Studies show that most people hit the keys much harder than necessary. Don't lift your hands far above the keyboard and bang your fingers down. Train yourself to use a softer touch and "drop" your fingers to reduce impact on the fingers and hands.

**Position fingers correctly.** Don't hold your fingers in awkward positions: crimped, stretched, or crumpled. Maintain neutral wrist position and arc fingers on a gentle, even curve.

**Keep relaxed.** Maintain good posture without tensing the muscles in your arms, fingers, neck, or back. Don't press your elbows in tight to your body.

forearms parallel to the floor or tilted slightly up. A thin profile also keeps you from having to bend your wrists back to type.

**Adjustable angle.** Adjust the angle so your wrists are flat and comfortable.

**Scooped (dished) keys.** Scooped key tops encourage your fingers to stay in the correct position.

**Moderate keystroke pressure.** Too firm an action requires extra force. Too sensitive an action can produce input errors and hand tension.

**Comfortable key spacing and layout.** Your fingers should rest comfortably without crowding. For those with larger hands, the keyboards of some portable computers may seem awkward. Layout should be familiar, and frequently used side keys (Shift, Return, and so forth) should be close to the main keys.

**Tactile or aural feedback.** Most keyboard users prefer feedback that indicates when they've made a keystroke.

# New Contenders for the Throne

Types of alternative input devices range from simple key layout rearrangements to sophisticated interpreters of voice input. Joining the revolution can be expensive: some alternatives initially cost well over 10 times as much as standard keyboards, but prices have been falling. Because there is no overwhelming evidence that the new alternatives are any safer, unless your present keyboard bothers you, wait for more scientific evidence before you switch.

If you decide to be adventurous, remember: Let the buyer beware! Be leery of unsubstantiated claims; it's best to try different designs, so make sure they have a money-back guarantee.

### Keyboards
Some of the new keyboard designs are merely changes in layout. Others are based on QWERTY, but offer new and variable geometry.

# The Dangerous Keyboard

*A standard keyboard can force your wrists into three unnatural positions. Exactly how and to what degree these positions contribute to injury is not known, but it has been suggested that by using less force in your typing (most people hit the keys far too energetically), you can lessen the potential damage to your body.*

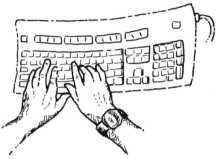

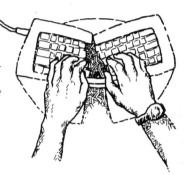

**Ulnar deviation.** *The wrists bend outward so the fingers can reach the keys. Ulnar deviation is alleviated in some new designs by splitting the keyboard so the key layout forms a V.*

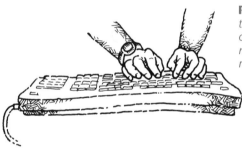

**Pronation.** *The wrists rotate the hands so they face downward, so the fingers can rest on the keys. Pronation is alleviated in some new designs by splitting the keyboard and raising the middle.*

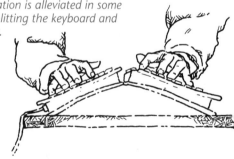

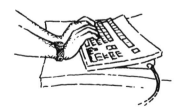

**Extension.** *The wrists tilt up (extend) to reach the keyboard. Use a wrist pad, adjust the keyboard's angle, or adjust your workstation so your wrist doesn't bend up or down. Make sure your wrist doesn't jab into any hard edges. Most experts suggest floating your hands while typing (see* **Shoulders to Hands***).*

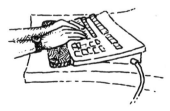

# Three Keyboard Safety Tips

Reduce your chances of injury from your keyboard in these three ways.

**Check height and tilt.** Make sure your keyboard sits at a height that keeps your forearms relatively parallel with the floor. Most desks are too high. Some experts suggest tilting the keyboard slightly away from you—propping up the front—to help level the wrists. (See **The Desk** and **The Perfect Workstation**).

**Consider a wrist rest.** Many people find that wrist rests help keep wrists and hands parallel to the keyboard. But improperly used wrist rests can do far more harm than good. Many experts suggest you should keep your wrists "floating" while you type, and use the pad to give your wrists a comfortable resting place between typing. Wrist rests should be thick and padded, and sit even with the keyboard (although some people prefer slightly higher), not below it. Try out wrist rests to make sure they fit your equipment.

**Use macros.** Use macros to decrease the amount of keying you do.

**Different key layout.** The Dvorak layout, developed in the 1940s as a faster alternative to QWERTY, runs a very distant second to QWERTY in popularity. The layout groups the most often-used letters where they are the easiest to press. Dvorak layouts have been shown to dramatically increase typing speed and accuracy, and are as easy to learn as a standard layout. But how a QWERTY layout reflects the rate of injury is unknown.

The Dvorak International Federation last collected statistics in 1984, at which time over 100,000 people were estimated to be using that layout. The Federation has no current statistics because of the wide dissemination through non-commercial sources of Dvorak-enabling software. Many keyboard manufacturers offer Dvorak layouts at little or no extra cost. And there is a wide variety of software—commercial, shareware, and public domain—to make your standard keyboard work with the Dvorak layout (then all you need are new key labels, and some learning time). Although you might type faster with a Dvorak layout, you may not be any less prone to injury.

## Different Geometries

Keyboards with angled sections designed to put less stress on the wrists and hands are now available from a number of manufacturers.

**EK1.** The EK1 keyboard from Somers Engineering represents the simplest type: at first glance it appears like a standard keyboard, but closer inspection shows that all the keys are set on a grid (like keypad keys) rather than staggered. According to the manufacturer, this allows the fingers to flex more naturally and reduces finger-to-finger interference when typing.

**Adjustable Keyboard.** Apple Computer's Adjustable Keyboard splits in the middle, allowing the two halves to be rotated apart to reduce ulnar deviation. The separate keypad can be freely positioned.

**Select-Ease.** Lexmark's Select-Ease keyboard's split sides can be rotated apart or separated completely. Cursor movement keys are provided on each half.

**FH101.** The FH101 from Fountain Hills Systems sets the standard keys in two separately angled bunches.

**MyKey.** The MyKey from ErgonomiXX appears similar to the FH101, but the two groups of keys pyramid
slightly in order to reduce pronation. MyKey's function keys are grouped in a circular pattern.

**MiniErgo.** The MiniErgo from Marquardt Switches
is an inexpensive V-shaped keyboard. A companion
moveable keypad is also available.

**Natural Keyboard.** The Microsoft Natural Keyboard contains key sections that are angled, split,
and rotated to encourage less stressful posture.
Three extra keys access Windows-only functions.

**Maltron.** The Maltron, the oldest design of the
group, places the numeric keypad between the two
scooped-out, separated halves of a dished layout.
Some of the ancillary keys have been moved more
radically—in some cases, to allow them to be pressed
by the thumb rather than the weaker little finger.

**Ergonomic Keyboard.** The Kinesis Ergonomic
Keyboard appears similar to the Maltron. The Kinesis
keyboard can be operated with one or two foot ped-
als. Kinesis claims that independent studies show its
keyboard reduces physiological stress and can be
quickly mastered.

**FlexPro.** The FlexPro Keyboard from Key Tronic (an
identical keyboard is made by ErgoLogic Enterprises)
splits the alphanumeric keys into two sections that
can be adjusted upwards and outwards.

**Comfort Keyboard.** The Comfort Keyboard System
from Health Care Keyboard Company represents the
most adjustable alternative. Each of the keyboard's
three sections can be tipped or rotated to any position the user desires. Sections can be rearranged, so
the keypad can be mounted on the left. The wide
range of adjustability allows the user to reconfigure
the keyboard from a standard, flat arrangement to a
more radical configuration in a series of steps.

## Radical Alternatives
More radical alternatives have already found favor
among the disabled, some of whom claim to have
been disabled by their standard keyboards. The
Americans with Disabilities Act has also increased

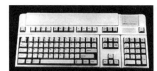
Somers Engineering EK1

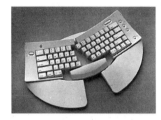
Apple Adjustable Keyboard

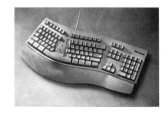
Microsoft Natural Keyboard

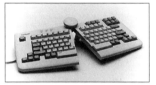
Lexmark Select-Ease

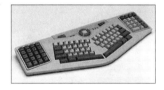
Fountain Hills Systems FH101

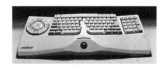
ErgonomiXX MyKey

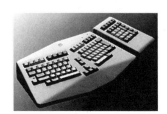
Marquadt Switches MiniErgo

*Maltron*

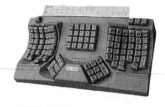

*Kinesis
Ergonomic
Keyboard*

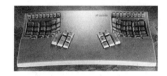

*Key Tronic
FlexPro*

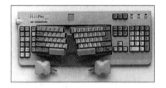

*Comfort
Keyboard
System*

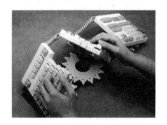

*DataHand*

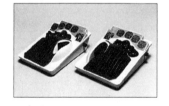

*Bat chord-key
input device*

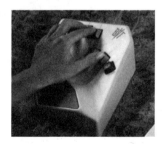

interest. The Act requires companies to accommodate disabled employees to a reasonable extent, including the purchase of specialized equipment (see *Resources*, below). It has been claimed (but not proven) that these low-stress alternatives can prevent injury. Beware that the immobility accompanying their use may cause its own problems.

**DataHand.** The DataHand system represents a unique attempt to reduce stress while keying. The user's fingers rest in wells that surround each finger with a number of magnetic switches, so typing (or mouse movement) is performed by moving the fingers slightly in one of five directions. A study done by an independent organization and paid for by the manufacturer showed significant pain reduction in people using the DataHand system.

**Chord keying.** Chord keyboards, like the Bat, are a relatively new class of input devices, and they possess significantly fewer keys than traditional keyboards—as few as six or seven. However, you can produce as many characters as a standard keyboard by pressing keys in combination, much like playing chords on a piano. Most chord-keying devices are designed to adjust to your hands with a minimum of stress. Their manufacturers claim they are surprisingly easy to learn and use. See **Where Else to Turn** for a listing of chord-keyboard manufacturers.

**Voice recognition.** Voice-recognition systems, until recently an expensive add-on for the disabled, are now readily available for the average user. The more sophisticated units are rapidly coming down in price; they can convert slow dictation into words. Less expensive alternatives can be utilized to trigger often-used functions, sometimes in conjunction with macro programs. See **Where Else to Turn** for a listing of voice-recognition systems.

## Pointing Device Pains

Are mice, trackballs, and other pointing devices less painful to use than keyboards? Which has the fewest risks? No one knows. Many people claim their mouse gave them a repetitive strain injury; but even though the world's mouse population is estimated at 60 million, there is just not enough and no conclusive research into the physiological effects of prolonged pointing device use to state many risks definitively.

However, one researcher, Pete Johnson—a graduate student at University of California Berkeley and San Francisco Ergonomics Laboratory—has compiled some information based on research and field observations. Some of the current knowledge is in his "Pointing Device Summary," which is available in electronic form (see **Resources**). (Much of the information in this section was adapted and condensed with permission from that source.)

While injuries at the computer may be due to a variety of causes (see **The Chair**, **The Desk**, or **The Perfect Workstation**), a number of body pains or discomforts may be related to identifiable aspects of mice or trackballs, or their use.

## Shoulder

Shoulder pain or discomfort may be due to postural problems caused by workstation setup or design, or to mouse use requiring repetitive movement of the upper arm. If you find yourself moving the mouse long distances, you might want to increase the mouse speed setting to reduce movement, but be vigilant for increased muscle tension. If you experience shoulder soreness, you may benefit from switching to a trackball. But if you do, watch out for three potential problems.

■ Trackballs use smaller hand and forearm muscles to produce movement, so you need to gradually work these muscles into shape to avoid stressing them. Don't switch to a trackball and use it intensively right away.

■ Most trackballs promote wrist extension (bending the wrist upward) by their design. Consider placing a foam pad in front of the trackball to reduce extension.

■ Trackballs use the thumb more than a mouse. Dr. Robert Markison, professor of surgery at the University of California/San Francisco School of Medicine, points out that the joint where the

# Good Pointing Techniques

Dr. David Rempel, Director of the Ergonomics Laboratory at University of California at Berkeley and San Francisco, suggests four ways to more safely move your mouse. Consider using these tips with other pointing devices as well.

■ Maintain a neutral wrist position.

■ Vary hand position throughout the day.

■ Don't press your hand into any hard edges.

■ Don't use force while clicking or dragging.

The following pointing device techniques may also prove helpful.

**Easy reach.** Make sure you can operate your pointing device without stretching your arm or putting your body into an awkward positions. Many keyboard trays may leave too little room for a mouse or tablet, forcing you to put the mouse on the desk, where it's difficult to reach.

**Don't tense.** Don't grip the device with too much force, a bad habit many mouse users fall into. Don't keep your arm constantly tensed while using the device, as this can tire the muscles and lead to injury.

**Let go.** Let go of the pointing device when you aren't using it to allow your hand and arm to relax.

# Pointing Device Design

Good pointing device design results in low stress on your body. Whether a new device fits your body and work style is best determined by test driving the device (though it is difficult in many stores, where they are kept packaged). However, the larger computer superstores often have hands-on displays for comparison. You should consider how the pointing device fits your body, its button activation pressure, and its movement requirements.

**Fit.** You must be able to hold a pointing device without putting too much pressure on your wrist, hand, or fingers. Some mice (especially the three-button variety) may be too wide for many hands. Others may be too small for large-handed people, forcing fingers into a cramped, claw-like contortion. Some trackballs may have sharp edges that are difficult to avoid.

**Activation pressure.** A pointing device button with high activation pressure may lead to problems with the tendons and muscles associated with finger movement. Find a device with low activation pressure—but not so sensitive you must keep your finger poised above it. Or consider using a trackball with a foot pedal.

**Movement factors.** You must be able to move a pointing device without putting your body into awkward positions or placing too much stress on the body parts required to move the device. Look for devices (or software for those devices) with variable tracking speeds.

thumb meets the wrist evolved much more recently than the rest of the hand skeleton, and is subject to wear. Make sure your thumb doesn't get sore from the trackball, and avoid trackballs that use the thumb to roll the ball.

## Button Finger

Fingers that activate buttons (and the fingers' associated tendons and muscles) may become sore due to button use or extensive mouse dragging. You might try using keystrokes when they can replace clicking, or try switching pointing device hands (but be aware that you may develop the same problems you had on the other limb). Or consider the following solutions.

If you think repeated button clicking gives you pain, you can try either a foot pedal or buttons that require less force. The Kraft Trackball can be used with foot pedal, but try it out before you buy it to see if it fits your body. Different mice have different button forces (both the old and the new Microsoft Mouse have particularly low activation pressures).

If repeated continual dragging seems to be your problem, you might want to try a drag-lock feature, which holds a "mouse-down" condition without continual pressure on the button. This may be a feature available with your mouse/software combination (as it is in three-button mice like the Logitech). An alternative for Mac users is a $3 shareware program called Power Clicks that remaps your mouse button to a keyboard key. Most trackballs also have drag-lock capabilities.

### Ring and Little Fingers

Your ring or little finger might develop pain due to incorrect pointing device size. Consider switching to a trackball or switching to different size of device. To reduce pain in the ring or little fingers, small hands may need to switch to a smaller device (like the original Microsoft Mouse), while large hands may benefit from a three-button device which is necessarily wider.

### Wrist

Some people use their wrists to move the mouse, keeping their arm immobile, which causes them to pick the mouse up repeatedly. These people may benefit from changing the mouse speed and moving the mouse more with their arm—but watch out for shoulder pain!

### Elbow

Pain around the elbow may be due to poor posture caused by improper workstation setup or design, or to repeatedly extending your wrist and fingers or constantly floating your fingers over the device in a fixed position. Consider a wrist rest to reduce wrist and finger extension. If you float your fingers over your pointing device, try to rest them gently on it to take some of the load off the tendons at the elbow.

> ■■■
> **The world's mouse population is estimated at 60 million**
> ■■■

## Resources

See **Where Else to Turn** for a complete list of companies, products, associations, and other helpful resources, including a list of alternative keyboards and input devices.

**Job Accommodation Network**. US (800) 526-7234; Canada (800) 526-2262. Information on Americans with Disabilities Act.

*The HAND Book*. Stephanie Brown (New York: Ergonome, 1993).

*Repetitive Strain Injury, A Computer User's Guide*, Emil Pascarelli, MD, and Deborah Quilter (New York: John Wiley & Sons, 1994).

*Pointing Device Summary Document*, Pete Johnson. Updated monthly on a Bitnet mailing list, C+Health. Subscribe by sending mail to the Internet mail address: listserv@iubvm.ucs.indiana.edu with the body of the message reading: "subscribe C+Health" followed by a space and then your first and last name (your e-mail address is automatically determined and should not be entered). If you have access to Usenet newsgroups, look for the group "bit.listserv.c+health".

# 12 The Perfect Workstation

## Positioning Yourself for Safer Computing

*Choose products based on what works the best, not what's cheapest.*

■ ■ ■

**The right equipment, adjusted correctly, provides one of the cornerstones of safer computing.**

■ ■ ■

## Related chapters:

- The Chair
- The Desk
- Keyboards and Mice
- Lighting

Your workstation should be designed and adjusted for your body and job to minimize physical stress, force, and repetition. Consider this chapter's contents as guidelines rather than hard and fast rules: they must be adapted to your situation. No workstation design can be guaranteed to be injury-free. Training, job design, schedules, and supervisory relationships need to be considered along with equipment in producing a healthy computing environment.

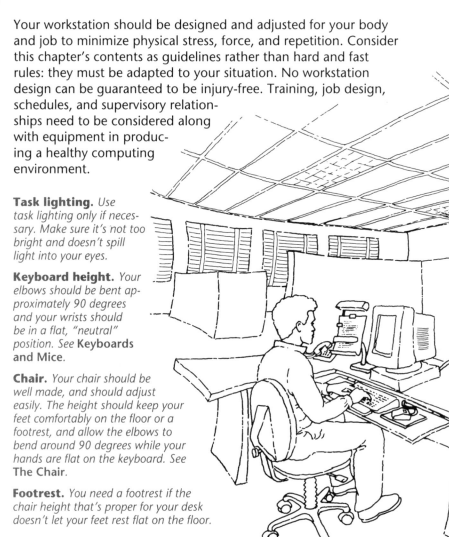

**Task lighting.** *Use task lighting only if necessary. Make sure it's not too bright and doesn't spill light into your eyes.*

**Keyboard height.** *Your elbows should be bent approximately 90 degrees and your wrists should be in a flat, "neutral" position. See* **Keyboards and Mice**.

**Chair.** *Your chair should be well made, and should adjust easily. The height should keep your feet comfortably on the floor or a footrest, and allow the elbows to bend around 90 degrees while your hands are flat on the keyboard. See* **The Chair**.

**Footrest.** *You need a footrest if the chair height that's proper for your desk doesn't let your feet rest flat on the floor.*

**Bright lights.** *Keep bright lights out of the field of vision. Orient your workstation to exclude light sources that can't be modified. See* **Lighting**.

**Ambient light.** *Indirect lighting is preferred; it shouldn't overpower the brightness of the screen. See* **Lighting**.

**Reflections.** *Control screen reflections by louvering or masking lights, repositioning the screen slightly, or attaching a glare shield. See* **Monitors**.

**Room surfaces.** *Use matte finishes and neutral tones to reduce brightness.*

**Noise.** *Music and office noise should not be loud enough to annoy or distract.*

**Air.** *Maintain a comfortable temperature, with adequate fresh air. See* **Office Air**.

**Adjacent monitors.** *If electromagnetic radiation concerns you, stay at least four feet away from the backs or sides of adjacent monitors (unless they meet MPRII guidelines). See* **Radiation**.

**Space.** *You should have enough space to adopt various comfortable positions. Your space should provide some privacy while allowing you to easily shift your focus to a distant object.*

**Work surface.** *Make necessary materials easily accessible. See* **The Desk**.

**Monitor.** *Ensure adequate resolution, keep it well maintained, and clean the surface regularly. See* **Monitors**.

**Monitor position.** *Traditional practice has been that the top of the screen should be at eye height or slightly below, but some experts now say a more downward gaze angle may be better. The monitor should sit at least 18 inches (45 cm) from the eyes, directly in line with the keyboard. See* **Lighting**.

**Electromagnetic Radiation.** *If you are concerned about electromagnetic radiation, place the monitor 30 inches (75 cm) away from you unless it meets MPRII (or stricter) standards. See* **Radiation**.

**Type size.** *The type displayed on your screen should neither be so small that it's hard to see, nor so large that it slows down your reading. See* **Monitors**.

**Keyboard.** *The keyboard should be slim, detached, and provide solid key-press feedback. See* **Keyboards and Mice**.

**Documents.** *If you refer to them often, keep documents on a copy stand adjacent to the screen.*

**Wrist rests.** *Some people find wrist rests helpful to maintain a neutral wrist position.*

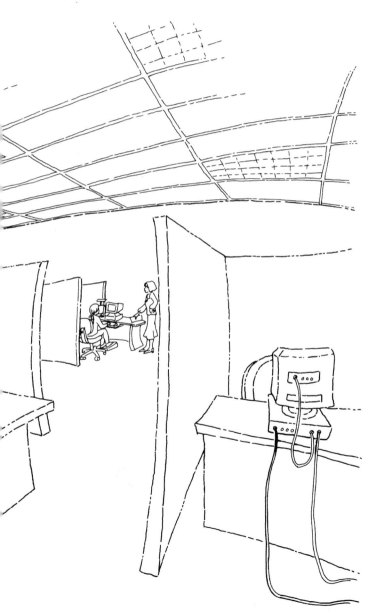

## Keep Moving

Prevent injuries that are caused by holding a static position for long periods. See **Schedules**.

- Shift your seated position frequently to remain comfortable Adjust your chair and workstation to accommodate.

- Take breaks and alternate tasks. Get up and move away from your workstation.

## Psychosocial Factors and Job Design

In addition to the physical factors that affect your work, you should also consider your supervisor, your job, and you.

**Your job.** Too much force and repetition should not be required by your job. The schedule and the other requirements of your job should not create undue psychological stress.

**Your supervisor.** Managers should be rewarded for keeping groups free of injuries. This can backfire if workers are discouraged from reporting CTD symptoms or are fired when showing early signs.

Stress expert Deborah Stiles points out that "stress greatly increases when the worker does not get along with his or her supervisor." Stiles suggests many ways a supervisor can ameliorate occupational stress: showing workers respect, trust, and concern; following fair disciplinary procedures; praising workers; expecting reaslistic performances; not monitoring every moment of a worker's activities; fostering good teamwork; and reducing task ambiguity or task conflicts.

**You.** You need sufficient training (and inclination) to adhere to safety principles. Talk to your supervisor about problems and see your health-care provider if they persist. Take proper breaks and consider stretching. Keep a positive attitude: lack of job satisfaction makes a worker more prone to suffer the deleterious effects of on-the-job stress. See **Schedules**, **Stress**, and **Stretching and Exercise**.

# Shoulders to Hands

### Carpal Tunnel Syndrome and Other Horrors

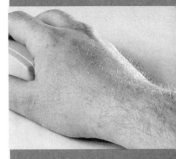

Computer work usually boils down to actions of the shoulders, arms, wrists, and hands. Because they're the critical link on the route from brain to screen, from thought to action, they suffer frequent abuse. All too often a computer user is stuck on automatic pilot, banging away at the keyboard, hell-bent on speed, working for hours on end in awkward positions. Such abuse has a painful toll according to *CTDNews*: millions of computer users suffer from cumulative trauma disorders (CTDs) of the shoulders, arms, wrists, and hands.

Cumulative trauma disorder is a term used to describe a range of injuries associated with long hours of repetitive movement. CTDs occur when overuse or misuse of the body is chronic, zapping the same body part or parts with repeating small traumas—an accumulation of wear and tear that can be painful and disabling. The condition can appear slowly or suddenly.

Both the ease of keystroking which lends itself to long periods of rapid and repetitive movement and the poor posture of many desk-sitters make computer users prime targets of CTDs. But you don't have to be a demon at the computer to suffer from injury. CTDs are often subtle affairs, developing slowly over time. Even light-strokers and short-stinters can eventually develop CTDs.

## Common Problems

CTDs can cause a variety of symptoms, and early symptoms can be hard to notice, so many computer users may not realize that problems are underway. When any of the following symptoms occurs (especially if it persists or becomes chronic), see a medical professional.

- Burning pain during noncomputer time, particularly during your normal sleeping hours

- Localized pain or dull achiness, with or without movement

*Cumulative trauma disorders are the fastest growing workers' compensation claim.*

■ ■ ■

**Awkward and static postures contribute to CTDs.**

■ ■ ■

## Related chapters:

- Stress

- Back and Neck Pain

- Keyboards and Mice

- Getting Help

- Radiating pain that travels up and down the arm or shoulder

- Numbness and tingling

- Weakness or stiffness

- Loss of muscle coordination or control

- Hands or arms tire more easily

> **...**
> **Static and awkward postures, and duration of keystroking are the main risk factors**
> **...**

With CTDs, it's common for several injuries to occur at once, causing multiple symptoms that may be tricky to pinpoint; weakness in one body part affects related body parts. Tingling in the hand, for example, could be related to a problem in the forearm. Or, pain at the elbow may be linked to the neck. Many specialists believe that psychological stress contributes to computer-related CTDs, since a common response to psychological stress is tensing muscles and tendons. (See **Stress**.)

## Muscles

Keystroking can't occur without muscle power from the upper back, arms, and shoulders. But overdoing it can strain and fatigue muscle fibers, often causing inflammation and soreness. Injured muscles are also prone to spasm—uncomfortable but not always painful. Although high force of muscle contraction may be related to developing CTDs, chronic muscle tensing with or without repetitive movement may be sufficient to cause injury.

Many computer users maintain postures that involve constant tensing of their neck, arm, and shoulder muscles, eventually impairing their efficiency. Stress leads to further tensing. Meanwhile, repetitive movements demand that the muscles perform. The stage is set for overworked muscles. Since blood nourishes and cleanses muscle tissue, poor circulation caused by static postures also contributes to muscle strain.

## Joints

Strong fibers called ligaments attach bone to bone, forming joints. Some joints are encased in a fluid-filled lubricating capsule that allows for a range of movement. Many computer users chronically overextend their arms, making them particularly vulnerable to joint problems at the shoulder and elbow. Once damaged, joints can become unstable and susceptible to recurring injury.

Some joints rely on bursae for cushioning. Bursae are fluid-filled sacs that help pad unprotected joints and unsheathed tendons from bone. Irritated tendons can irritate and inflame adjacent bursae, a condition called bursitis. Bursitis commonly occurs near the shoulder joint, causing pain and impaired movement. (There's

# Physiology of Carpal Tunnel Syndrome

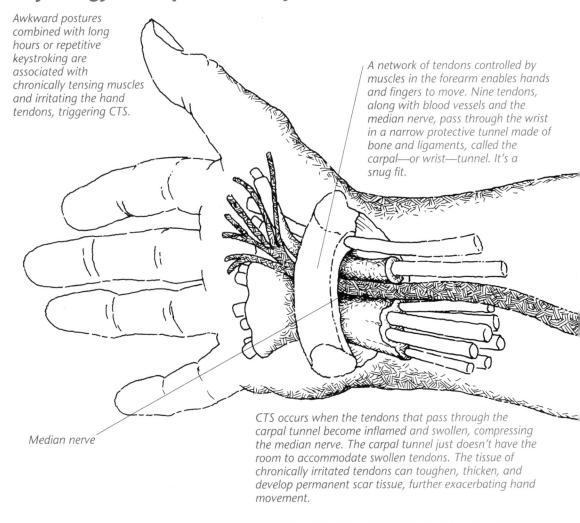

*Awkward postures combined with long hours or repetitive keystroking are associated with chronically tensing muscles and irritating the hand tendons, triggering CTS.*

*A network of tendons controlled by muscles in the forearm enables hands and fingers to move. Nine tendons, along with blood vessels and the median nerve, pass through the wrist in a narrow protective tunnel made of bone and ligaments, called the carpal—or wrist—tunnel. It's a snug fit.*

Median nerve

*CTS occurs when the tendons that pass through the carpal tunnel become inflamed and swollen, compressing the median nerve. The carpal tunnel just doesn't have the room to accommodate swollen tendons. The tissue of chronically irritated tendons can toughen, thicken, and develop permanent scar tissue, further exacerbating hand movement.*

controversy among specialists as to whether computing aggravates existing cases of bursitis, causes new ones, or both.)

## Tendons

Tendons connect muscles to bones. When muscles tense, tendons and their sheaths can become irritated. Chronically tensing or straining muscles and tendons can lead to tendinitis, a painful irritation and inflammation of the tendons, or to tenosynovitis, an inflammation of the tendon sheath.

73

# Will You Develop a CTD?

It is impossible to say who will develop a cumulative trauma disorder, but some people are more at risk than others. Watch out for these factors associated with CTD development.

**Poor posture.** Awkward postures put uneven stress on body parts, leading to myriad problems, particularly of the back and wrists (see *Pay Attention to Posture*).

**Poor typing technique.** Typing with twisted or cocked wrists or forearms not parallel to the floor can cause strain. Letting your wrists or forearms rest on a surface while you type may overwork and stress the muscles in your hands. Pounding the keys puts stress on the fingers. See **Keyboards and Mice**.

**Stressful job circumstances.** Demands of the job like deadlines (newspaper reporters) or repetitive typing tasks (data-entry people) are associated with developing CTDs. Office environment factors, like crowding or noise, can increase psychological stress in some people, which is also associated with CTD development. See **Stress**.

**Nature.** Your body's particular physiology may predispose you to certain CTDs, and diseases like alcoholism and diabetes can also be contributing factors. Pregnancy is known to increase the chances of developing carpal tunnel syndrome. See **Pregancy**.

**Lifestyle.** Poor diet, lack of sleep, and smoking can all be risks for developing CTDs. See **Health Basics**.

**Tendinitis.** Tendons located near joints are particularly prone to tendinitis, because they're often unsheathed or unprotected. The most common CTD, tendinitis, is marked by localized tenderness or achiness, swelling, shooting pains, and pain with arm movement. Tendon strain is also associated with sudden or severely awkward movements.

In the arms, many kinds of tendinitis are associated with computer use.

- Flexor tendinitis, which affects the tendons on the inside of the arm and hand, is caused by chronically flexing the fingers down from the wrists.

- Extensor tendinitis, which affects the tendons on the outside of the arm and hand, is caused by chronically extending the fingers up and back from the wrists.

- Tennis elbow (lateral epicondylitis), which affects the outside of the elbow is often associated with repetitive, jerky motions of the arms.

- Golfer's elbow (medial epicondylitis), which affects the inside of the elbow, can be caused by bending the wrist while rotating the forearm.

- Rotator cuff tendinitis, which affects the tendons at the shoulder joint, can be caused by working with a constantly raised elbow.

**Tenosynovitis.** Tendons often run through lubricating fluid-filled protective sheaths, called synovial sheaths; the lubricating fluid is called synovial fluid. Repetitive movements sometimes cause the accumulation of excess synovial fluid, a condition called tenosynovitis. Symptoms of tenosynovitis include swelling, pain with movement, redness and pain to the touch. De Quervain's disease is a tenosynovitis that affects the thumb region. It's associated with constantly extending the thumb to reach the spacebar. Tenosynovitis of the flexor tendons contributes to a condition called carpal tunnel syndrome, discussed below.

## Nerves

Nerve pathways travel from the upper spine to the fingers. Problems anywhere along the route can trigger symptoms, often elsewhere. Nerve irritation in the neck, arms or shoulders, for example, can cause symptoms in the hands and wrists. Severe nerve problems can cause permanent, disabling damage (see **Back and Neck Pain**).

The most common nerve problem for computer users is carpal tunnel syndrome (CTS). Ulnar nerve problems also can occur from computer use. The ulnar nerve, which runs down the arm to the wrist, is particularly vulnerable to irritation at the elbow. Often this irritation occurs at a particular location, the cubital tunnel, and so the condition is called cubital tunnel syndrome. Cubital tunnel syndrome is linked to constantly pushing the elbow against hard surfaces, such as armrests or desk edges, putting chronic pressure on the ulnar nerve.

■ ■ ■
**Problems in one area often trigger problems in another.**
■ ■ ■

**Carpal Tunnel Syndrome.** Although it occurs less frequently than many other computer-related CTDs, carpal tunnel syndrome (CTS) gets more attention. CTS is so notorious largely because, like other nerve-related CTDs, it can be highly debilitating—advanced cases can leave permanent nerve damage, severely limiting hand movement and coordination. Some CTS sufferers lose their ability to use a keyboard, and have to change careers. CTS was also one of the first CTDs widely reported by computer users.

The good news is that when caught early, treatment combined with changes in computing behavior can reverse the course of CTS.

CTS occurs when the median nerve is entrapped in the carpal tunnel (see *Physiology of Carpal Tunnel Syndrome*, page 73). Symptoms of CTS include pain, numbness, and tingling in the hands, particularly in the first three fingers and the thumb. The same symptoms can appear in the forearms, often at the same time as in the hands.

CTS also causes burning pain in the wrist during time away from the computer, particularly in the middle of the night—even to the point of waking up some sufferers. Night burning and numbness are among of the best diagnostic indicators of CTS.

Preexisting conditions, such as arthritis or scar tissue from prior hand or wrist injuries, may exacerbate CTS; they can also make exact diagnoses difficult. Pregnant women are more vulnerable to

## Thoracic Outlet Syndrome

The thoracic outlet is a triangular region located above the shoulder between the collarbone and the neck. Blood vessels and nerves serving the arm pass through this area. There's some controversy among specialists about the impact of computing on the thoracic outlet, but many believe that some computer users develop postures that chronically compress the nerves and blood vessels in the region, triggering neck tension, shooting pains, tingling, and numbness down the arm.

CTS due to edema, or fluid retention, which often occurs with pregnancy (see **Pregnancy**). Low thyroid activity, diabetes, and other illnesses may contribute to CTS, as can a pinched nerve in the neck or thoracic outlet region.

## Wise Treatment

Start by admitting you have a problem. Many computer users resist admitting to work-related pain or discomfort, feeling they can overcome or ride out symptoms on their own. This is a dangerous attitude. Long-term untreated problems can cause permanent and painful disability.

Occasional or mild CTD symptoms may disappear with rest and the use of over-the-counter anti-inflammatory pain relievers (such aspirin or ibuprofen). Many people find relief by icing or using alternating hot and cold water baths. But when experiencing acute or recurring symptoms, self-treatment isn't advised. Arm or wrist splints and slings, arm rests, wrist rests, and other apparatus advertised as preventing or treating CTDs can further damage an existing problem if they aren't used properly.

Let a medical professional—preferably with a background in CTDs—guide your treatment (see **Getting Help**). Doctors can employ a variety of specialized tests to aid accurate diagnoses of CTDs. Specific problems usually require specific treatments, making medical diagnoses critical. Treatments range from surgery to anti-inflammatory medications or injections (see **Medications**) to physical therapy to simple rest.

## Take Precautions

Preventive measures reduce the likelihood that any computer-related CTD will occur. Many arm and shoulder problems can be prevented or minimized by following a few guidelines. Depending on the job or nature of the computing work, some will be easier to adhere to than others. Try to incorporate as many into your work routine as possible.

## Work Defensively

Prevent wrist and hand problems from occurring with these methods.

- Create diversity in your work tasks to avoid long periods of time in the same movement. Take frequent rest breaks from repetitive keystroking. (See **Schedules**.)

- Consider an ergonomically designed workstation. (See **The Perfect Workstation**.)

- Try warm-up or break exercises and stretches. (See **Exercise**.)

- Watch out for pushing or resting wrists or forearms against hard desk edges; this can compress nerves and cause nerve problems.

- Pay careful attention to the positioning of the keyboard. Train yourself to use light keystroking to avoid force. (See **Keyboards and Mice**.)

- Stay warm. Working at cold temperatures may increase the chance of developing CTDs.

## Straighten Those Wrists

Constantly flexing and extending the hands up and down by bending the wrists is believed to be a major contributor to CTS and other hand and wrist problems. Do whatever it takes to keep the hands flat and even with the wrists and forearms. This is best achieved through proper positioning of the desk and keyboard. Also avoid constantly stretching the hands side-to-side from the wrists. Keep hands straight.

## Be Mindful of Mouse Movements

Any movement that's repeated over and over, including gripping, pushing, or clicking a mouse, can injure related body tissues. When using a mouse, try to avoid overstretching the fingers or thumbs. And don't extend your pinkies. Keep the mouse in easy reach from the keyboard, and be gentle; don't grab or tap the mouse forcefully. Mouse users should avoid extending or flexing their wrists. Keep wrists even with the hands and forearms. Try a trackball or other alternative (see **Keyboards and Mice**).

## Splint's Value in Preventing CTS Questioned

Dr. David Rempel of the University of San Francisco recently discovered that the flexible splints often worn by workers to prevent or postpone carpal tunnel syndrome don't seem effective. Rempel measured the pressure on the carpal tunnel of splinted and unsplinted workers performing a repetitive task. The pressure on the carpal tunnel rose about the same amount in all the workers, leading Rempel to question the efficacy of splints as protection. "Basically the study shows the splint has no value in reducing carpal tunnel pressure and may increase the risk in some people," said Dr. Rempel.

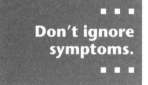

Don't ignore symptoms.

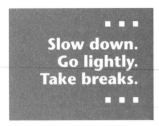

**...
Slow down.
Go lightly.
Take breaks.
...**

### Pay Attention to Posture

Don't slouch forward or round your shoulders. Sit in a comfortable position that evenly distributes weight over your spine, while supporting your lumbar curve. Arms should extend comfortably from the elbow so that hands can use the keyboard without bending up or down at the wrist. Avoid bad resting habits, such as leaning your forearms or wrists on the desk or arm rests. Frequent leaning can compress nerves, causing nerve damage and impaired muscle functioning. Bad posture often develops in childhood or over long periods of time and can be very difficult to correct. Try to maintain a periodic awareness of your body throughout the day.

### Don't Be A Creature Of Habit

Most computer users develop idiosyncratic posture-related work habits—pressing the forearms into the desk edge, tilting the head towards the window, keeping one arm mostly on an arm rest, tucking the left hand between the thigh and the chair, drooping the chin into the chest. Anytime the body does the same thing over and over, day after day, it stresses and strains the involved body parts, potentially leading to—or exacerbating—CTDs. It's much safer to move around a lot and change positions frequently, keeping the body lively and active, and not set in its ways.

## Resources

See **Where Else to Turn** for a complete list of companies, products, associations, and other helpful resources.

***The Carpal Tunnel Syndrome Book.*** Mark A. Pinsky (New York: Warner Books, 1993).

***The HAND Book***. Stephanie Brown (New York: Ergonome, 1992).

***Repetitive Strain Injury: A Computer User's Guide.*** Emil Pascarelli and Deborah Quilter (New York: John Wiley and Sons, Inc., 1994).

# Back and Neck Pain

**From Annoying to Agonizing**

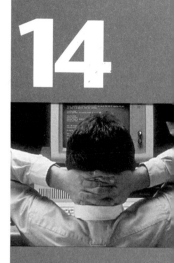

Many people don't realize that sitting stresses the back and neck; the longer you sit, the more the strain. Bad postures are particularly taxing. Add to this reaching out and moving your hands, eyes glued to a screen, and you immediately increase the likelihood for neck- and back-related pain. Overstressing the muscles, nerves, tendons, and joints used in computing can create a recurring state of body tension often called static overload. Time sitting at a computer can aggravate existing back problems or prompt new ones, and often it's not clear which is occurring.

With back and neck pain, it's important to keep in mind that the torso is a system of interrelated parts. A myriad of symptoms in the arms, legs, head, and chest can indicate back or neck problems, including numbness, tingling, sharp pains, burning, spasm, vague aches, soreness, lack of muscle strength, and stiffness. When nerves at the spine become pinched, irritated, or compressed, the entire nerve pathway can be affected. Pain or tingling in the foot, for example, may mean nerve damage in the spine. All this makes for tricky diagnoses.

## Problem Areas

Beware compression. People who sit for extended periods—such as an average work day in front of a computer—are particularly vulnerable to problems resulting from downward pressure on the spine. Hours of staying in one position, arms extended over a keyboard while you crane your neck to view a screen, increases the pressure on the disks and puts loads on tendons, muscles, and nerves. Additionally, forcing muscles into tensed positions for long hours leads to generalized muscle fatigue. Muscle spasm is often the body's response to an underlying problem, such as a torn ligament or irritated nerve.

*A myriad of symptoms can indicate back or neck problems.*

■ ■ ■

**For every moment of sitting upright, hundreds of muscles are hard at work, fighting gravity.**

■ ■ ■

**Related chapters:**

- Shoulders to Hands
- The Chair
- The Desk
- Schedules

# A Look at the Back

*An interrelated bundle of important bones, muscles, and nerves shares the enormous burden bestowed on the computer user's back. Spinal compression is one of the most common problems affecting computer users.*

## The Spine

*Delicately sculpted for strength and flexibility, the spine supports muscles while housing the spinal cord, which branches off to form the peripheral nervous system—the intricate pathway of nerves that transmits messages between the brain and the rest of the body.*

## Muscles and Ligaments

*A variety of muscle groups stretch across, underneath, and on both sides of the spine, supporting the back while contributing to the movement of the arms and hands. Thousands of ligaments hold the system together.*

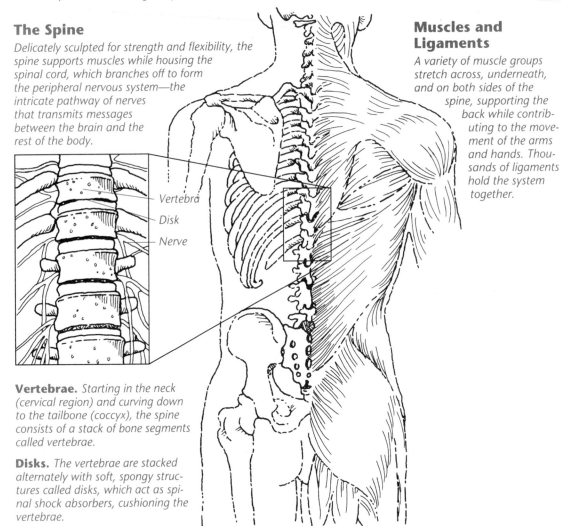

Vertebra
Disk
Nerve

**Vertebrae.** *Starting in the neck (cervical region) and curving down to the tailbone (coccyx), the spine consists of a stack of bone segments called vertebrae.*

**Disks.** *The vertebrae are stacked alternately with soft, spongy structures called disks, which act as spinal shock absorbers, cushioning the vertebrae.*

**Spinal cord.** *The spinal cord, connecting the brain to the body, travels along the spine in a tunnel-like protective hollow at the rear of each vertebra.*

**Nerves.** *Smaller nerves exit from the spinal cord through holes on either side of each vertebra, spreading to the rest of the body.*

## Don't Lose the Curves

Healthy back posture allows the spine to maintain its natural S-curve. When standing, the pelvis usually tilts slightly forward, with the center of gravity over the lumbar curve (the inward bend at the small of the back), evenly distributing weight to establish equilibrium. Walking takes even more pressure off the spine. Sitting, on the other hand, tends to tilt the pelvis backward, flattening the lumbar curve. This results in uneven and increased pressure on spinal disks. Hour after hour of rounding the shoulders and holding the head forward—off the center of gravity—puts extra stress on the upper spine.

## Running Out of Fuel

Inactivity, or sitting for long periods, slows blood circulation, decreasing the efficiency of muscles. When slowed circulation is combined with demands on the muscles, lactic acid (a by-product of muscle activity) may accumulate, causing muscle fatigue. (Muscle fatigue can also result from overexercising.) Since computing requires muscle power but doesn't provide much heart-pumping exercise, computer users are vulnerable to the aches and soreness of muscle fatigue.

## Squashing Thighs

Blood circulates through arteries and veins. Sitting can squash major veins located on the back of the thigh, pressing them against the seat of the chair. When these veins are compressed for prolonged periods, the flow of blood through them slows; the veins can also swell and become irritated and painful.

# What To Do

If you experience acute pain, chronic pain, numbness, tingling, or any changes in urination or bowel function, see a doctor. Many back problems creep up slowly, worsening with time, so proper diagnosis is essential for relief and healing.

A few simple steps may help relieve mild or occasional symptoms. And preventive measures can go a long way.

# The Tricky Tailbone

Sitting for long periods of time can irritate the tailbone, or aggravate an already injured tailbone. The tailbone, which serves no purpose to the body's functioning, is the last vertebra of the spine, tapering downward to form a point. Hard surfaces are particularly irritating.

Pain from coccyx injury varies from mild to severe, depending on the injury's severity. If sitting is a necessity, use a spongy chair seat, or cushion your seat with a doughnut-shaped cushion or fluffy pillows. Injured tailbones heal, but it takes time.

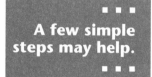

**A few simple steps may help.**

81

## Be Neck Aware

The neck can be an elusive factor in computer-related pain, because problems in the upper spine can cause symptoms in the hands and arms, such as tingling and numbness, with or without pain in the neck or back. In other words, your neck may feel fine, but your hand could be numb and tingly due to pressure on the spinal nerves. Doctors treating computer-related injuries see two significant neck problems.

■ Tension neck syndrome, marked by stiffness, muscle spasm, and radiating pain, can be caused by chronic neck-muscle strain. Sitting and constantly staring at a screen places particular demands on these muscles, which must tense to keep the head balanced over the spine, face forward, and chin up. Maintaining this position for long periods can lead to this painful condition.

■ Double-crush syndrome refers to a condition that occurs when the nerve is pinched in two places: one at the neck (or a little farther down, in the thoracic outlet) and the other down in the hands or wrists. A nerve pinch in one of these places alone may not cause symptoms. But the two nerve pinches combined may aggravate the entire nervous system of the hands, arms, shoulder, and upper back.

Reduce the chances of neck injury with the methods suggested for the back. And keep your chin slightly tucked in; avoid stretching the neck out or up. Avoid activities requiring twisting, jerking, or repetitively bending the neck, such as reading from papers far from the keyboard or crooking a phone between your shoulder and cheek. Use a headset or a document stand.

**Start with the chair.** Increasingly, office chairs are designed with back health in mind. Adjust them properly and often. Regularly changing positions and postures is one of the best ways to avoid overtaxing the back and neck. A reclined position is easiest on the back (but hard on the neck), so recline as much as you can as long as your neck is supported. This can be tricky for many computer users, but detachable keyboards can help. In all seated positions, maintain your lumbar curve. Use the back of your chair to support your lower back; don't sit forward and lean over, as this tends to further decrease the lumbar curve. Sometimes placing a rolled-up towel or pillow in the small of your back helps. Try to sit so that your feet are flat on the floor or a footrest. Avoid rounding your shoulders. See **Chairs**.

**Continue with the workstation.** The position of the keyboard and screen play a major role in the activities of the neck, arms, legs, hands and shoulders—all linked to the back. Keep the computer screen directly in front of you; keep reading material within comfortable sight, at eye level or below; and keep telephones within easy reach or use a headset. See **The Perfect Workstation** and **The Desk**.

**Take active breaks.** At break time, don't stay in your chair. Take pressure off the spine and get the blood pumping by moving around. Walk around the office, jump up and down, go outside for fresh air. See **Schedules**.

**Shift positions now and then.** From the chair to the desk, adjust your workstation periodically. Try not to fall habitually into one computing position. Even small changes help avoid overtaxing certain muscles or parts of the spine. If possible, alternate between sitting and standing; increasingly, work-places are accepting standing as a viable computing posture.

**Consider pain medication.** Mild or occasional back pain may be relieved by using over-the-counter pain medicines such as aspirin or ibuprofen. But pain is your body's way of saying, "Stop"; so if pain persists, see a doctor.

**Practice back safety everywhere.** Whether in the office or at home, protect your back. Squat to pick up heavy loads and use leg muscles when lifting. Get exercise; regular physical activity aids blood circulation and strengthens muscles. Strong torso muscles help support the spine. Walking is an excellent exercise for the back, easy on the spine. Watch your posture; don't slouch, stand with shoulders back, head high, letting your back curve naturally, tilt your pelvis forward, stomach tucked in, and don't lock your knees. If prolonged standing is necessary, put one foot on a stool or thick phone book.

## Resources

See **Where Else to Turn** for a complete list of companies, products, associations, and other helpful resources.

**Texas Back Institute**. (800) 247-BACK. Will answer questions and provide material about back problems.

*Treat Your Own Back*, Robin McKenzie (Waikanae, N.Z.: Spinal Publications, 1988).

*Treat Your Own Neck*, Robin McKenzie (Waikanae, N.Z.: Spinal Publications, 1988).

# Advances in Diagnosis and Treatment

Medical diagnosis and treatment of back problems has always been an uphill battle. Studies show that up to 85 percent of back pain cannot be diagnosed definitively, so—not surprisingly—effective treatment has often proved elusive. Luckily, most back pain resolves itself. But for those unlucky enough to suffer a serious problem, advances in diagnostic and treatment techniques hold promise.

Both MRI and CAT scans can image soft tissue, including nerves, giving doctors a much better view of possible problems in the back than was available with older X-ray techniques. Although relatively recent advances, MRI and CAT scans are increasingly accessible, and doctors have worked with their results for long enough to increase their efficacy in diagnosing back problems.

For those requiring back surgery, new, less invasive procedures may be available. If you need back surgery, be sure to ask your doctor about new arthroscopic techniques (where instruments are inserted through small incisions) which may decrease both complications and recovery time.

# 15 Stress

## It Can Work for You or Against You

*Chronic stress is linked to a range of health problems.*

■ ■ ■

**Fight or flight among high-rises and asphalt.**

■ ■ ■

**Related chapters:**

Long ago, when we wandered the earth as hunters and gatherers, our response to danger was to fight, or take flight. The perception of danger triggered a rush of hormones, prompting a physiological reaction to aid strength, speed, and alertness, often called the "fight or flight" response.

Now we're creatures of high-rises and asphalt, but our bodies have the same physiological response to demands. The ring of a telephone or an impending deadline makes hormones rush, hearts beat faster, and blood flow with extra speed. This is stress, and it can help us meet challenges, but it can also lead to crippling physical and psychological damage. Social interaction with managers and peers, job instability, time pressures, performance standards, even boredom take their stressful toll. Computer work is a potential culprit in the onslaught of office-related stress.

### Stress Overload

Each person responds differently to outside demands (often called stressors). But for most people, a little stress, off and on, is a positive, energizing stimulant. In fact, boredom can itself be a damaging stressor. The trouble begins with too much stress, when the body stays on constant alert, hormones surging like an open faucet.

Chronic stress may be linked to a whole range of health problems—some serious—including heart disease, high cholesterol, hypertension, ulcers, exhaustion, anxiety, and depression. Less serious but potentially debilitating conditions linked to stress include head-, back-, and neckaches; insomnia; upper respiratory infections; and skin rashes such as psoriasis and eczema.

### Stress in the Computer Workplace

Office work, in general, is chock-full of potential stressors—from flickering lights and jarring noises to deadlines and demanding bosses. Computer workers face additional sources of stress: monotonous keyboarding; hours of staring at the screen; lack of social interaction; lack of physical movement; lack of autonomy, independence, or control over work; and, increasingly, monitoring technology designed to electronically track computer work and send the information to supervisors.

Because everyone reacts differently to stress, a stress level appropriate for you may be inappropriate for a co-worker; the trick is finding a healthy balance between positive, motivating stress and stress overload. Preventing stress overload starts with paying attention to symptoms and taking steps to reduce stress and relax. In many cases, work can be made less stressful; even small changes can help.

## Stress Statistics

Stress is a well-known culprit in damaging the health of computer users.

- 75 to 90 percent of visits to primary care physicians are for stress-related ailments.

- In 1992 and 1993, 26 million workers in the US were under surveillance on the job.

- Costs to industry from job stress exceed $150 billion a year.

- Many states and provinces have laws regulating the length and number of breaks, including lunch, that workers are entitled to. Consult your state health department.

- A 1990 study by Johns Hopkins University found that the occupations with the highest number of workers suffering from depression included secretaries, typists, data entry keyboarders, and computer equipment operators.

## What to Do

Stress is accumulative—a reaction to demands from all areas of life, on and off the job. Therefore, preventing stress means focusing on the home and the workplace. Some people have an easier time cutting back on work-related stress than others, depending on the nature of the job and the style of management. In some cases, changing occupations or

## The Body's Reaction to Stress

Normally, the body's reaction to stressors is short-term or intermittent, lasting long enough to fuel a response; then things quiet down. Chronic stress occurs when the body stays on constant alert.

Demands from the outside world are perceived as threats or calls to action. In response, the adrenal glands pump out two hormones, cortisol and adrenaline. They raise heart rates, blood pressure, and blood flow. Simultaneously, blood sugar is diverted from internal organs to the brain to increase alertness.

After the danger passes, the brain triggers the release of a variety of substances (including endorphins) that perform a number of different functions that includes inhibiting adreneline and bringing the body back to a more relaxed state. Chronic stress occurs when cortisol and adrenaline levels stay high, keeping the body in a state of constant alert.

# Heed the Warnings

At some point or another, most people experience many of the early symptoms of stress overload for short periods without serious consequences. But increases in the frequency or intensity of symptoms, including chronic problems, may indicate a need for medical attention. Watch out for the following symptoms.

- Frequent headaches
- Frequent back-, neck-, or other aches
- Recurring heartburn or acid indigestion
- Bursts of rapid heartbeat
- Sleep disturbances
- Increased bad moods or anger
- Constant tension; feeling wound up or on edge
- Unusual lethargy, exhaustion, or apathy
- Hives or skin rashes
- Increased drug or alcohol use.

places of work may be the best solution. But several things are worth trying first.

Bear in mind the three Rs: relaxation, reduction, and reorientation. Stress management should be a combination of reducing exposure to stressors, relaxing—quieting the stressed-out body—and reorienting expectations and self-demands.

## Make Wise Use of Breaks and Lunches

Break for several minutes each hour and wiggle your fingers, take your eyes off the screen, stand up and stretch. On longer breaks, do what makes you feel good: Chat with co-workers, get fresh air, find a quiet place to shut your eyes, or jog around the block. Everyone's different; tap into what lifts your spirits. (See **Schedules.**)

## Good Eating

Start with a healthy breakfast. After a night's rest, the body thrives on morning fuel; eat carbohydrates for long-lasting energy. Light, nutritious lunches and frequent healthy snacks—nuts, fruit, crackers—are better energizers than large meals eaten less frequently. And drink plenty of fluids throughout the day, but watch out for dependence on caffeine or sugary soft drinks; they may be linked to moodiness.

## Build Bits of Physical Exercise into Your Work Day

Take the stairs instead of the elevator. Park your car in the far corner of the parking lot. Take the bus. Walk to someone's desk instead of using e-mail. Find a place in the office to exercise at breaks. Encourage your co-workers to join in. Develop a lunchtime exercise regime. Ease tension with simple stretches and relaxation exercises done right at the desk. (See **Stretching and Exercise.**)

## Plan Ahead

Schedule to meet deadlines. Use planning to avoid stressful work back-ups and overloads. Take as much control in your work schedule as the job allows.

## Talk It Out

Get work frustrations off your chest by talking about them with family and friends. Share feelings with co-workers, but avoid workplace gossip that may come back to haunt you—and even increase your stress levels by amplifying frustrations. Otherwise, talking can be an excellent way to release bottled-up feelings. Many larger businesses have counselors on staff, who are experts in job stress. Make use of them.

## Fight Monotony

If you are feeling bored and restless, look for ways to make your work more challenging—much easier to do in some jobs than others. Ask for more responsibility, ask to learn new technology, brainstorm new ideas with co-workers, consider switching to another department. Many people fear change, but mastering new challenges can be tremendously invigorating and breaks monotony. Take the first step.

## Consider Alternatives

Some companies offer ways to personalize or tailor the work schedule, such as flex time and job sharing. Some even allow for leaves of absence to take classes or to do volunteer work or community service. Breaking routine can reduce stress.

## Go to Management

If job stress becomes a major concern, it may be time to discuss larger changes, either on an individual level or office-wide. Take note of sources of stress that may be affecting large numbers of employees. Approach your supervisor, union representative, or a manager you're comfortable with. Try to stay calm, prepared to negotiate, with ideas and suggestions for change. Of course, these suggestions might not work in all corporate cultures. You know your company better than I do. You might have to proceed with caution. (See **Changing the Workplace**.)

> ■ ■ ■
> **The trick is finding a healthy balance between positive, motivating stress, and stress overload.**
> ■ ■ ■

# Resources

See **Where Else to Turn** for a complete list of companies, products, associations, and other helpful resources.

**National Institute of Mental Health**, Office of Scientific Information, 5600 Fisher Lane, Parklawn Bldg., Room 7-103, Rockville, MD 20857. (301) 443-4513. Free materials on depression, psychological stress; referrals to professional organizations, not doctors.

**Association for Applied Psychophysiology and Biofeedback**. (800) 477-8892. Will supply local referrals for professionals who may specialize in CTDs and who incorporate biofeedback into their practices.

# 16 Schedules

## Taking Proper Breaks

MBER
T W T F S
1 2 3 4
6 7 8 9 10 11
13 14 15 16 17 18
20 21 22 23 24 25
27 28 29 30 31

JANUARY
S M T W T
2 3 4 5 6
9 10 11 12 1
16 17 18 19 2
23 24 25 26
30 31

*More frequent but shorter breaks are beneficial.*

■ ■ ■
**Most people don't break often enough or long enough.**
■ ■ ■

**Related chapters:**

- Stress
- Software
- Changing the Workplace

A classic theory of management (McGregor's "X Theory"), suggests that if allowed, employees will try to take as many breaks as they can. For typical computer workers, the opposite has been observed to be true. They don't take enough breaks; instead they continue to sit at the computer until they have some type of pain or discomfort that forces them to stop.

Computer work is static and constrained, the modes of interaction are limited, and there is a small range of postures available—all factors that tire muscles quickly. You can prove this yourself; if you try to sit bolt upright in the correct posture, it feels good for about five minutes. But because the muscles are in continuous tension, circulation is cut off and lactic acid builds up, producing pain and finally forcing you to change your posture.

Experts now feel that the traditional schedule of morning and afternoon work periods, each divided with a 15-minute break, is outdated. While those traditional breaks may serve useful purposes—going to the bathroom, socializing, getting a snack—they aren't frequent enough to allow the body to recover from the stress related to computer work. A more frequent but shorter break schedule increases productivity and decreases discomfort, but there is no exact formula for the perfect work/rest schedule.

## New Ways to Work

There is a dangerous misconception among many managers that increasing break time decreases productivity. A recent NIOSH study tested a work-break regime designed in response to studies that suggested breaks should occur more often than every hour, and that muscle tension needs to be alleviated even more often. NIOSH tested a schedule of three-minute breaks every 40 to 50 minutes, with 30-second micro-pauses every 10 minutes. The study compared that schedule to the traditional schedule of midmorning and midafternoon breaks.

On breaks, users were told to do something other than work at their computers. The results of the study showed a decrease in worker discomfort—and a significant increase in productivity.

## How Much and How Often

Dr. Robert A. Henning, a psychology professor in industrial organization at the University of Connecticut, says that computer users don't break early enough, often enough, or long enough. All break schedules should meet the following criteria.

**Breaks need to be taken in advance of pain.** If you break after you feel discomfort, it will take much longer to recover than if you take a break earlier.

**Breaks need to be long enough to allow recovery.** Spontaneous breaks are often only five to 10 seconds—not sufficient to allow for recovery from strain.

**Breaks need to be taken often enough.** Muscle stress recovery needs to go on throughout the working day to maintain low stress levels.

### Recommended Regimens

While authorities differ as to how often and how long computer users should pause for breaks, most have upped the recommended numbers over the past several years.

- The Occupational Medicine Clinic at San Francisco General Hospital recommends a 10-minute break (or alternate work) at least once an hour, and a computing day of four to six hours.

- US West and AT&T reduced CTD symptoms by providing one-minute "mini-breaks" every 20 minutes.

- The British Association of Scientific, Technical, and Managerial Staffs recommends a 30-minute break after a maximum stretch of two hours at the keyboard (furthermore, they advise no more than four hours of computer work per day).

## Gentle Reminders

Breaks often come at inopportune times, so they are easy to ignore and forget. See **Software** for some computer-based systems that can help you remember to take breaks.

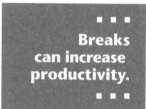

. . .
**Breaks
can increase
productivity.**
. . .

# What to Do on Your Breaks

Use breaks to shift your position, stretch, exercise—anything to use your muscles differently from regular computer work. And remember that breaks aren't the only way to let muscles recover from static and constrained postures.

- Vary tasks so computer work is interspersed with other activities.

- Place equipment like printers far enough away so you get up and walk to them.

- Have a snack or something to drink.

- Catch up on your professional reading.

- Neaten up your office.

- Take a moment to relax.

■ NIOSH has recommended a 15-minute break for every two hours of moderately demanding VDT work (or for every one hour of intensive VDT use). The positive results of the NIOSH study discussed earlier—and the results of a study involving two insurance companies using a similar regime—suggest that the schedule of a three-minute break every 50 minutes with 30-second breaks every 10 minutes is also effective. The efficiency of the insurance companies' claims processing was higher during the test period than in a typical earlier period without the regime.

■ In his book, *Repetitive Strain Injury: A Computer User's Guide*, hand expert Dr. Emil Pascarelli suggests, "If you are not injured, take a 5- to 10-minute break from typing for every half hour that you work. One break per hour should include stretching: the other should be spent doing nonkeyboard activities."

# Office Air

## Bad Air, Computers, and Disease

Buildings can make you sick. Some buildings do not adequately circulate their air, so particles and gases given off by the furniture and the inhabitants can accumulate, increasing infections, headaches, allergic reactions, and eye, nose, and throat irritations. Computers don't cause this phenomenon of indoor air pollution, called sick building syndrome. The most common offenders include insufficient general ventilation, dust, and mold in your heating and ventilation system, and gases released by carpets, fabrics, and wall coverings. But computers may make a few aspects of your air even worse.

## How Computers Make Things Worse

An invisible climate streams around your computer. The screen, cooling fan, and the heat of various components all modify the circulation of gases and particles in the air near your computer, potentially leading to a number of health problems. If you experience any of these conditions, and they lessen or disappear over the weekend, it might suggest that the office air is worth investigating; if you suspect that your office building has a case of sick building syndrome, see *Resources*, page 93.

**Facial dermatitis.** There is an increased incidence of facial dermatitis (reddening, itching, prickling of the face) among people who sit in front of computers. One of the likely causes is the dust and particles propelled toward the face by the electrostatic field of the video screen. The problem is worsened by the low humidity present in heated buildings in the winter.

**Red and sore eyes.** Three aspects of the desktop computer can cause red, burning, and itching eyes: its heat dries the air, its fan blows air which may evaporate lubricating tears, and its screen

*Your computer can increase some of the effects of sick building syndrome.*

■ ■ ■

**An invisible climate swirls around your computer.**

■ ■ ■

**Related chapters:**

- Monitors

# Computer Microclimate

*The air around the computer swirls with invisible activity.*

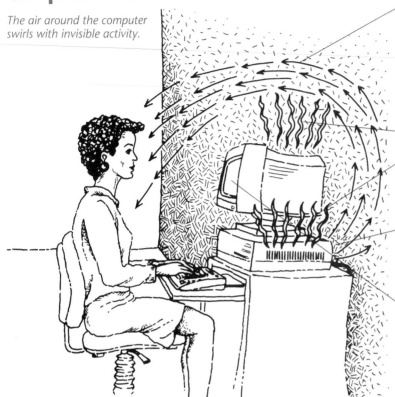

**Dust movement.** *The electrostatic field of the screen attracts negatively charged particles toward the screen, creating a film of dirt and repelling positively charged particles toward the operator's face.*

**Heat.** *Heat builds up in the various electronic components, drying the air and causing convection currents around the computer.*

**Fan.** *Most computers direct the exhaust away from the operator, but it can be redirected toward the face by adjacent surfaces.*

**Ion depletion.** *When negatively charged particles hit the screen, they are neutralized, so negative ions are depleted from the immediate area.*

creates an electric charge which propels particles into the eye. Eyes that are fatigued from straining to see are particularly susceptible. See **Eyestrain**.

**Nausea, stress, and fatigue.** Some people believe that nausea, stress, and fatigue are just three of the conditions that can be attributed to negatively charged particles in the air. Although the vast majority of scientists lend no credence to those claims, everyone concurs that computer screens attract and neutralize negatively charged particles around them, vastly reducing the number of negative ions in the air.

## What to Do

A few simple measures may alleviate airborne annoyances around your computer.

**Check the air system filters.** Office air often gets dirty, stale, and moldy when the filters in the air system aren't cleaned regu-

> ■ ■ ■
> **Try increasing moisture and decreasing dust.**
> ■ ■ ■

larly. Check with maintenance to see if cleaning or changing the air filters isn't the key to cleaner air in your office.

**Increase moisture.** Most people are comfortable with a relative humidity level of around 50 percent. A humidifier can increase moisture, but exercise caution: some computer equipment does not like high relative humidity, and humidifiers can harbor disease-causing fungus and bacteria.

**Keep the air flow away from your face.** Even if you regard it as a cooling breeze, make sure that the airflow from the computer's fan is not redirected toward your face.

**Decrease dust and particles.** Make sure the office is vacuumed and dusted often. Periodically have the dust cleaned from inside your computer.

**Decrease static.** Carpets can be treated with fluids to decrease static electricity. Check to ensure that your keyboard (like those available from most major manufacturers) has a grounded conductive surface to reduce your body's static charge.

**Add ions.** If you are a positive believer in negative ions, you may want to add an ion generator; there is one designed specifically for sitting over the screen (see *Resources*). Keep in mind that significantly more research would be necessary before it could be proved that adding negative ions makes office air healthier. For the present, this is a theory not supported by science.

## Resources

See **Where Else to Turn** for a complete list of companies, products, associations, and other helpful resources.

**National Institute of Occupational Safety and Health (NIOSH)**. (800) 356-4674.

Air-quality consultants, found in local Yellow Pages under **Environmental Engineers**, can measure office air.

## Ozone Alert

Many laser printers and photocopiers produce ozone, a gas molecule comprising three oxygen atoms, unlike the oxygen gas molecule normally found in the air, which has two oxygen atoms. At low levels, ozone irritates the eyes, nose, and throat and may trigger allergies; at high levels it produces nausea and headaches. Ozone-producing equipment contains ozone filters which should be replaced every 12 to 18 months, or perhaps sooner if they become clogged due to large amounts of dust in the environment. It's recommended that this equipment be located in well-ventilated areas. Your nose detects ozone well. Ozone can often be smelled (you may have noticed its sour odor before a storm) even when it is present in amounts considered too low to be dangerous. However, recent research suggesting that extremely low levels of ozone may trigger allergies. If you're concerned, consider turning off your laser printer if you won't be using it for the next two or three hours. Recently, some copier and laser printer equipment manufacturers redesigned their products to emit significantly less ozone.

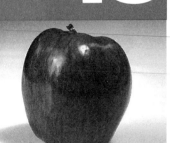

# 18 Health Basics

## Health-Conscious Living and Work Benefits

*Remember to use common sense at the keyboard.*

. . .

**Out-of-shape computer users are more vulnerable to muscle strains, aches, and pains.**

. . .

**Related chapters:**

- Stress
- Stretching and Exercise

Your parents told you that a proper diet, regular exercise, plenty of sleep, and time spent relaxing can make you healthier. What they probably didn't tell you is that those common-sense practices can significantly contribute to your health as a computer user by reducing the possibility of injuries, and reducing the effects of those problems that do occur.

Applying common sense and a few widely accepted guidelines for good health can help to bolster strength, stamina, and a sense of well being, making a significant impact on how you feel in all aspects of your life, including when you're at the keyboard.

## Get Regular Exercise

Just sitting at the computer uses thousands of back, neck, torso, arm, and leg muscles, requiring a steady blood supply for fuel. Regular exercise improves cardiovascular fitness and builds muscle strength, which increases muscle efficiency and helps to prevent strain. Regular exercise is also associated with improving overall energy level, mood, and self-esteem.

Specialists recommend heart-pumping exercise—running, walking briskly, swimming, bicycling—at least three times a week, for at least 20 minutes. If it's been a while since you've made your body work, ease into an exercise regime slowly. For suggestions on exercises you can integrate into your workday, see **Stretching and Exercise**.

## Get a Good Night's Sleep

Chronic sleep disorders are extremely common, affecting millions of people. Sleep problems can be short or long term, and for many people, once the sleep cycle gets knocked out of whack, worrying about sleep exacerbates the problem. It can be difficult to break this cycle.

But relief is possible. If you can't fall asleep, or wake up in the night and can't get back to sleep, you should get out of bed, go to a different room, and find a relaxing but engaging activity: reading, working a crossword puzzle, writing, or taking a bath. Then, when you start to feel drowsy, go back to bed.

Don't drink alcohol to try to make yourself sleepy. Alcohol has a high sugar content; once the sugar kicks into the bloodstream, it can wake you up. Avoid caffeine after about three p.m. Try ear plugs or a sleep mask to block noise and light. For occasional insomnia, over-the-counter medicines may help, but don't make them a habit.

Excessive sleeping is often a symptom of depression, anxiety, or stress overload. When any sleeping difficulties are chronic, consult a doctor.

## Take Time to Relax

Most computer work involves stress, and chronic stress is linked to a variety of mental and physical health problems (see **Stress**). Since most jobs don't allow for much opportunity for deep relaxation, make it a priority off the job. Give yourself as much "down time" as possible to make up for the hours of "on time" demanded at work.

Regular exercise, massage, and meditation are proven relaxants; you probably have your own. Incorporate as many of them into your regular routine as possible.

## Eat Properly

> ■ ■ ■
> **Chronic sleep disorders are extremely common, but relief is possible.**
> ■ ■ ■

Increasingly, healthy eating is linked to long-term health benefits, including illness prevention. Our daily diet also affects how we feel. A balanced diet that's low in fat and high in fruits, vegetables, and grains gets top marks from most nutritionists. Start each day with a solid breakfast; morning fuel is essential to getting the body up and running after slumber. Eat lunch to power afternoon activities, but don't overdo; enormous meals can cause drowsiness. And don't skip meals. This can lead to stomach pains and lethargy.

Snack wisely. Avoid empty calories. Carbohydrate-laden foods—bread, pasta, whole grains—provide long-burning fuel, filled with vitamins and minerals. Nuts are nutritious, but high in calories. Fruits and vegetables and popcorn (without butter), are healthy low-calorie snacks.

Sugar, on the other hand—a major ingredient of candy bars, doughnuts, and many snack foods and soft drinks—is used up quickly and supplies almost no nutrients.

## Office Effects of Unhealthy Habits

Most people don't need to be reminded about the dangers of cigarette smoking, or alcohol or drug abuse. In addition to being linked to long-term health problems, excessive smoking, drinking, and drugs can affect how you feel each day—even if you don't touch the stuff in the office. Many larger businesses offer confidential employee assistance programs to help break addictions, so don't be afraid to ask about them. For people who must seek help from an outside source, many organizations, hospitals, and clinics provide excellent services.

If you're trying to lose or gain weight, consult a doctor first. Many diets aren't nutritionally balanced and will affect your daily energy level and mood. Drink plenty of fluids, but don't rely on the caffeine found in coffee, tea, and many soft drinks to charge your day. Yes, caffeine enhances alertness, but this can backfire; too much can lead to caffeine dependence, associated with mood swings and headaches.

## Check in Now and Then

Blood pressure, cholesterol levels, and weight are a few things that can help gauge health. Have these checked periodically—every couple of years, or more often if you have a known concern. Occasional monitoring can help identify problem areas before they become life-threatening.

# Stretching and Exercise

## Improving Health and Preventing Injury

*Sitting too long can injure you.*

The human body didn't evolve to sit; it functions best when it stands or walks. Sitting can slow circulation, produce muscle aches, and contribute to back and neck stiffness. And years of sitting day after day can lead to much more dangerous conditions, such as heart disease and spinal problems. To perform well, the body needs to regularly move through its natural range of motion—keeping joints lubricated and muscles toned.

Exercise is not a panacea—a National Institute of Occupational Safety and Health (NIOSH) office study showed that passive breaks improved mood and comfort as much as breaks incorporating exercise. And exercise breaks should not be seen as a complete solution to office health; they are only one aspect of the office ecosystem. But there is no question that exercise can improve health and mood. Although office work may seem designed to keep you from moving your body, with a little effort your workday can become part of an overall fitness program.

■ ■ ■

**Never stretch to the point of pain or discomfort.**

■ ■ ■

## Integrated Exercise

Aerobic exercise can be incorporated into your workday. Try to develop an attitude that seeks ways to exercise muscles in different ways. Here are a few tips.

**Use the stairs.** Stairs are a great way to improve cardiovascular performance and stamina.

**Park about a five-minute walk away from the office.** Or, if you live less than a few miles from work, consider walking. Brisk walking is a great way to start your day and loosen up on the way home.

**Run errands at lunch.** Maybe not run, but walk quickly. See how much you can accomplish in a limited period, but don't get stressed out!

**Related chapters:**

- Health Basics
- Stress
- Software

97

**Integrate exercise throughout your workday.**

**Exercise other muscles during time off.** A few parts of your body can get more than enough exercise at work. Use leisure activities to exercise your neglected muscles, instead of straining those that are overworked. Swimming and jogging are generally good alternatives for a computer user.

## References

See **Where Else to Turn** for a complete list of companies, products, associations, and other helpful resources.

"A review of physical exercises recommended for VDT operators," **Applied Ergonomics**, Vol. 23, No. 6, December 1992. NIOSH review of the usefulness and safety of 127 office exercises.

**Sitting on the Job: How To Survive the Stresses of Sitting Down to Work**, Scott Donkin (Boston: Houghton Mifflin Company, 1989).

**Stretching**, Bob Anderson (New York: Random House, 1980).

## Before You Begin

Exercise isn't for every body.

**Think.** Start slowly. Not doing any exercise is safer than overdoing it when you are out of shape. Listen to your body; never stretch to the point of pain or discomfort. Use your common sense as to what you can do safely.

**Think twice.** Stretches or exercise can worsen some cumulative trauma disorders, even incipient problems you are unaware of. To be safe, check with a doctor to ensure that stretching or exercise is right for you.

**Think thrice.** Many doctors recommend checkups before beginning an exercise program, especially if you've had recent surgery or haven't exercised regularly for some time.

# Work Warm-Ups

*Stretching before work can prevent muscle strains by preparing your body for the demands of sitting and working the keyboard. You can also warm up as you change tasks throughout the day.*

## Posture Stretch

*Sit straight, maintaining a lumbar curve.*

*Reach both arms straight up, as high as you can, while imagining a rope pulling your head straight up.*

*Allow arms to slowly drop into your lap, and relax your neck.*

*Repeat five times.*

## Back Stretch

*Stand straight, and clasp your hands together, placing them in the small of your back.*

*Push your hips and hands forward, arching your body.*

*Immediately come back to the upright position.*

*Repeat five times.*

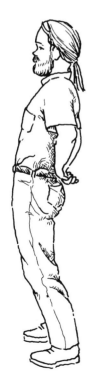

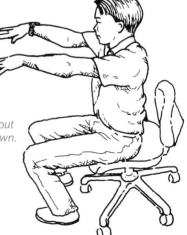

## Finger Stretch

*Hold your arms straight out in front of you, palms down.*

*Spread the fingers apart until you feel resistance.*

*Hold for five seconds, then relax.*

*Repeat five times.*

# Desk Stretches

*You might include these stretches as part of your daily tasks—but be sure to also regularly get out of your chair. Each stretch can be performed in sets of up to five repetitions, depending on comfort and time.*

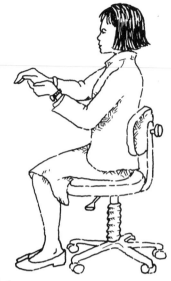

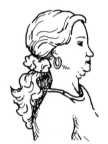

### Neck

*Sit straight, eyes looking straight ahead.*

*Pull head back, creating a double chin.*

*Hold for a few seconds.*

### Hands and Wrists

*Hold left hand in front of you with palm facing up.*

*Place palm of right hand onto the fingers of left.*

*Using your right hand to provide resistance, try to press the fingers of left hand up.*

*Switch hand positions and repeat.*

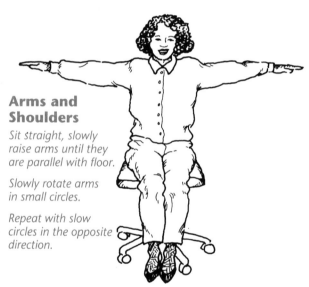

### Arms and Shoulders

*Sit straight, slowly raise arms until they are parallel with floor.*

*Slowly rotate arms in small circles.*

*Repeat with slow circles in the opposite direction.*

### Legs and Ankles

*Stretch one leg out and up*

*Move foot around in two complete circles*

*Repeat in other direction.*

*Repeat with other foot.*

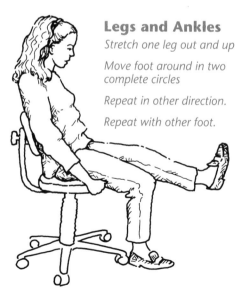

## Look Away

Every 10 minutes look away from the screen and focus on the most distant object available for 10 seconds. This should be done just once, not in repetition.

# Medications

### Use with Caution

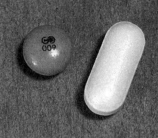

Sometimes computer work causes pain. Headache, eyestrain, and cumulative trauma disorders may have you reaching for over-the-counter medications. In more extreme cases, you may find relief with medications only available with a doctor's prescription.

Medications can be a valuable and welcome relief for computer-induced pain, but they must be used wisely. Many are powerful drugs with potentially serious side effects. And unless you use them rarely, most medications represent only a temporary or partial solution for a computer-related health problem. Investigate the office environment and your computing routine to determine what is causing your pain, and then solve the problem at its source.

## Over-the-Counter Pain Relievers

It is a common misconception that the government allows drugs to be sold over the counter because they are safe and not as potent as prescription medications. Aspirin, ibuprofen, and other nonsteroidal, anti-inflammatory drugs (NSAIDs), and, to a lesser extent, acetaminophen, can be as effective as many prescription-only pain relievers. In fact, so much so that they are often prescribed by doctors.

But these medications can also be dangerous. Both aspirin and ibuprofen have a number of side effects—most commonly stomach irritation, a problem that varies widely among individuals. Aspirin and ibuprofen can also cause ulcers, kidney damage, and adverse effects on the liver. Acetaminophen, although easy on the stomach, can cause a fatal overdose with the ingestion of relatively small amounts. If you are currently taking a prescription drug, on a diet prescribed by your doctor (low-salt, low-sugar), pregnant, or nursing, you should check with your doctor before taking any over-the-counter pain relievers. And check the labels of any other

*All pain relievers have possible side effects.*

■ ■ ■

**Use the right pain reliever.**

■ ■ ■

**Related chapters:**

- Health Basics
- Stress
- Back and Neck Pain
- Shoulders to Hands

**101**

# Warning

All of the drugs listed in this chapter can have serious side effects. In most cases these problems are rare, but since the list is as long as your arm, it is only practical to list a smattering of them. These drugs can be potent, so use them with good sense.

- Follow your doctor's instructions and any directions that come with the medication.

- If you have a question about medication, ask a pharmacist or your doctor.

- Some of the medications in this chapter cause drowsiness. Make sure they are not affecting you adversely before you try to drive a car or engage in other potentially dangerous activity.

- The information in this chapter relates to adults only. Children have special requirements when taking any medication. Consult a doctor if you have concerns.

drugs you are taking, to make sure you aren't taking the same thing already (many over-the-counter drugs include a mix of different pain killers).

If you find yourself taking an pain reliever day after day without a doctor's supervision, it should signal the need for another approach. First, all of these medications are potentially dangerous with long-term use. Second, it indicates a chronic problem that needs fixing in some more effective way.

## NSAIDs (Aspirin, Ibuprofen)

The nonsteroidal, anti-inflammatory drugs (NSAIDs) represent some of the most successful drugs available. They are inexpensive, yet can effectively relieve pain, inflammation, and swelling. If you find you can't tolerate one NSAID, there is sufficient variety available that another may work for you.

Many people get upset stomachs (and a few can develop ulcers) from taking NSAIDs; aspirin is considered slightly worse than ibuprofen in this regard. To ease stomach irritation, take these medications at mealtime or with a glass of milk, or dissolve the tablet in a glass of water. Buffered aspirin, touted to be easier on the stomach than normal aspirin, actually isn't. Coated aspirin does cause less stomach irritation, but instead can irritate the lower intestine and takes longer to work. In rare cases NSAIDs (especially ibuprofen) can cause kidney damage, which often goes unnoticed in early stages, and so can result in kidney failure. Also in rare cases, NSAIDs can cause liver effects, including abnormal enzyme levels.

## Acetaminophen (Anacin-3, Tylenol)

Acetaminophen (commonly found under the brand name Tylenol) is a triumph of marketing. When first introduced, the entrenched makers of NSAIDs felt acetaminophen was little threat: it had no anti-inflammatory action and wasn't as effective a pain reliever (although it did have fewer side effects). But the consumer now sees it as being analogous to aspirin.

If you can't tolerate NSAIDs, then acetaminophen is the over-the-counter pain reliever of choice. It is easier on the stomach than NSAIDs, but not completely benign, so you may want to take it at mealtimes or with milk. Because of the potential for liver damage, you shouldn't take acetaminophen for over 10 days without a doctor's approval.

Think twice about drinking alcohol while taking acetaminophen (especially if you regularly drink alcohol), as you might be increasing your risk of liver damage. And taking high doses of vitamin C prevents your body from excreting acetaminophen, which could lead to liver and kidney damage.

## Prescription-Only Medicines

Although your doctor may prescribe an over-the-counter medication, there are a number of other choices for more specific intervention.

### Muscle Relaxants

Your doctor may prescribe muscle relaxants if you are having muscle spasms, muscle tightness, or problems sleeping because of pain. A common first choice of muscle relaxants is Flexeril. It is in the same class of drugs as tricyclic antidepressants and will often help people sleep better.

Common side effects of Flexeril are drowsiness and dizziness; they can be severe enough in some people to force them to stop taking it. Flexeril can also lead to water retention and dryness of the mouth. The latter can result in increased tooth decay if you don't brush and floss well. It is advised that you do not drink alcohol while taking this medication.

### Steroids

Steroids reduce inflammation and swelling. They are usually given through injection, most often in the wrist for carpal tunnel syndrome or in the elbow for tendinitis. In other cases they are given orally over a one- to 10-day period.

Steroid injections are most beneficial when they are made to the precise location of the injured tissue, but they can harm tendons when administered incorrectly; make sure your doctor is experienced. Although the injection itself is usually not very painful, a common side effect is increased pain for several days, before the pain is reduced. Occasionally, a white or purplish mark (about the size of a quarter) will appear at the injection site due to depigmentation of the skin. Although in some instances the discoloration can be permanent, it usually fades with time. Less commonly a loss of fatty tissue can alter the appearance of the site of the injection.

## Mind over Pain

Drugs are not the only method of controlling pain. Many people are able to reduce their pain through relaxation exercises and pain-control techniques. If you can't or don't want to take medications, ask your doctor for alternatives.

## Vitamin B₆

Vitamin B₆ has been suggested as an effective remedy for carpal tunnel syndrome and other cumulative trauma disorders. At this point, its efficacy is questerioned by many doctors. And the vitamin is toxic in high doses.

### Antidepressants

If you have chronic tension headaches, if you are unfortunate enough to be suffering chronic pain from severe injury or disability, or if you're are having sleep difficulties, your doctor may prescribe antidepressants. Antidepressants may help pain for two reasons. First, because you could very well be depressed; and, second, because there are lots of studies to show that some of the antidepressants actually help control pain.

A common side effect of tricyclic antidepressants (the most often prescribed) is drowsiness. Constipation can also occur, which can be helped by increasing fiber in the diet. Sometimes people experience a sour or metallic taste.

While taking tricyclic antidepressants, you should avoid alcohol and large quantities of alkaline food (for example, milk products, most vegetables except corn and lentils, almonds, and most fruits).

### Narcotics

For severe pain, a doctor may prescribe a narcotic, such as codeine. A doctor may also prescribe a low dose for patients with ulcers or who cannot tolerate NSAIDs.

Although narcotics can be very effective for short periods, they can be habit-forming with prolonged use, so most doctors will avoid long-term prescriptions except in special circumstances.

Narcotics cause drowsiness and may cause a false sense of well-being. Be sure you react well to them before driving or engaging in other activity where you need to be alert. Constipation is a common side effect; relieve it by eating more foods with high fiber content (fruits, leafy vegetables, and grains).

## Resources

***The Aspirin Handbook: A User's Guide to the Breakthrough Drug of the 90s***, Joe Graedon, Tom Ferguson, and Teresa Graedon (New York: Bantam Books, 1993).

***The American Medical Association Guide to Prescription and Over-the-Counter Drugs***, Charles B. Clayman, editor (New York: Random House, 1988).

# Kids 21

## Concerns about the Computer-Age Child

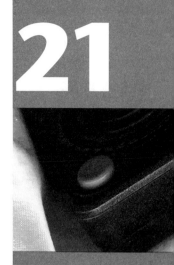

As a writing tool, learning aid, and vehicle for fantasy, the computer has taken up residence in playrooms and classrooms. As many adult computer users are well aware, kids can be some of the best computer experts around. But computer-active children are vulnerable to the same computer-related ailments as adults, and, with children, psychosocial factors of computer use may play a particularly important role.

While computers can have a positive impact on learning and skill development, they may also prompt social isolation and reduce physical exercise. And many video games expose youngsters to violent and sexist themes. The keys to being a responsible parent are: knowing the software, being aware of how your child is using the computer, and stepping in when the situation demands it.

## The Joy of Computers

Computers have been shown to have positive effects on children.

### Skills and Success
Research shows that computers can help youngsters develop hand-eye coordination and problem-solving skills. In addition, computer games offer opportunities for success—high scores and winning—to kids who can't participate in or aren't comfortable with sports.

### Education
Educational software has made some marvelous contributions to teaching, providing appealing alternatives to the textbook and the chalkboard. Special software adds new possibilities in teaching educationally disadvantaged and physically disabled youth.

*Children are vulnerable to the same computer-related ailments as adults.*

■ ■ ■

**Computers in the classroom and at home have led to young, sophisticated computer literates.**

■ ■ ■

**Related chapters:**

- Health Basics
- Shoulders to Hands

Children learn and create by doing, and a computer is a good tool to help them. But parents should be involved in their children's computer use, just as they are involved with their schooling and television watching.

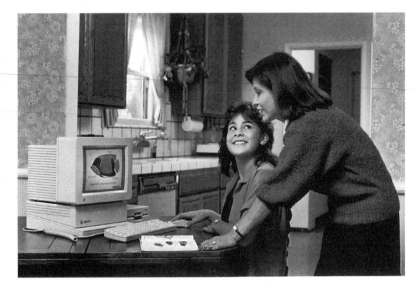

### Tools for the Future

Kids who use computers gain valuable skills that help prepare them for future careers. Early exposure to computers can provide a powerful jumpstart in the work force.

## Did You Know

■ Computers are installed in 52 percent of elementary and secondary classrooms in the United States.

■ Research shows that playing arcade-sized video games (the stand-up kind) provides about as much cardiovascular exercise as a brisk walk.

■ For many kids, computer time is in addition to television time, extending the overall amount of time in front of a screen.

## When to Step In

Some aspects of computer use may require a little monitoring. Here's when to step in.

### Screen Potatoes

Computer games can give the illusion of play, complete with shouting and jumping up and down, but most of the action takes place on the screen. A child's fingers and eyes may get some exercise, but the rest of the body barely moves; computer use isn't an adequate source of aerobic or cardiovascular exercise. Limit weekly computer time, particularly noneducational use, and don't let the computer supplant vigorous play. Bear in mind that games are designed to keep a child's attention, so it may be difficult getting them to take a break.

## Violence and Sexism

War, fighting, killing, and destruction are repeating themes in video games. It's often good guys versus bad guys, but winning is measured by damage done—the more the better. Sex roles tend to be stereotypical, with aggressive men, male creatures, or male animals battling evil and rescuing passive maidens. Some researchers believe that exposure to these themes can influence behavior, making children more prone to violence or sexism. Others believe that children screen out content and are able to distinguish between reality and media.

The video-game and computer-game industries recently developed separate rating systems to inform parents about the potentially offensive content of their products. While the video-game system has met with general approval, critics have charged that the computer-game rating system lacks impartiality and is difficult to understand.

If this issue concerns you, review video games and software; most manufacturers have 800 numbers—printed on boxes or available through directory assistance—for questions about their products. Make use of them.

## Just Me and My Floppy

By and large, using a computer is a solo event, whether studying math with educational software or piloting a spaceship in a video game. Kids who spend a lot of time doing either may be spending a lot of time alone. Some computer games and programs are designed for partners or teams, but many aren't. Playing and studying with peers teaches valuable social skills in compromise, negotiation, and cooperation. So watch for antisocial behavior; don't let your child hide in the computer. And don't sacrifice social time for computer time—aim for a healthy blend.

## Money Talks

Each day computers and software become more accessible and less expensive. But they're still luxury items, which many people can't afford. With so many kids having access to computers at home and in schools, children without access may be vulnerable

> ...
> **Kids need to be taught healthy computer use.**
> ...

## Epilepsy Caution

A recent study by Dr. William Graf at the Children's Hospital and Medical Center in Seattle, Washington, confirmed that some children experience epileptic seizures while playing video games. While there are still few children who are susceptible, the number may be larger than was generally recognized. There's no evidence that video games cause epilepsy; rather, the games can trigger seizures in people who are photosensitive: susceptible to particular visual stimuli like flashing lights or flickering images. Parents of children with epilepsy are encouraged to check with their doctors about photosensitivity.

to feeling left out, insecure, and inferior to their computer-comfy peers. Overemphasizing computers adds to the pain of inequities; keep them in perspective. Encourage kids to understand that computers are simply tools. Vibrant thinking, feeling, and acting can and does take place without them.

### Just Like Mom and Dad

With children, as with adults, pay attention to lighting, posture, and long hours of repetitive movement that may be taxing wrists, hands, and fingers. Many games involve repetitive and forceful movements— the kinds of movements that can lead to cumulative trauma disorders. Although children may be protected from injury by their natural tendency to change position frequently, those who sit statically for long periods need the same preventive measures as adults.

### Modem Madness

Many computers today are bundled with modems (or you may buy one separately). If you allow your child access to it, make sure he or she is not abusing it. There is a wealth of bulletin boards out there— hundreds in some cities—and it is difficult to monitor what information (like pornography) your children are accessing.

# Software 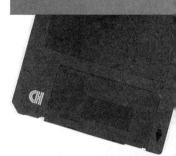 **22**

## Safe Computing Assistance

Computer sorcery: Being transformed into a mindless servile drudge by the instant gratification provided by your computer. Characterized by transfixed vision, static posture, and long periods without breaks, it results in anxiety, eyestrain, repetitive strain injuries, and other complaints.

Sound familiar? A proper computer work schedule, exercise program, and a health-conscious attitude are sometimes not enough; you may need to shatter your computer's spell before you can exercise your eyes, stretch, or get up and take a break.

A few software packages are available that automatically display exercise programs and, at appropriate intervals, suggest healthy alternatives to sitting in front of your mesmerizing screen. Most of these packages are integrated programs to reduce eye, musculoskeletal, and psychological stress; others have more specific roles. Additionally, a number of utility programs can be drafted to help you compute safely. Keep in mind that research has not yet proven many benefits from exercising at the keyboard (see **Stretching and Exercise**). However, taking frequent breaks improves productivity and decreases the risk of injury (see **Schedules**).

## Spectrum of Healthy Software

Many of the health-related software packages share similar features, including exercise programs, advice on workstation setup and posture, and various safety checklists. Vision Aerobics is the only computer-safety package designed specifically for the eyes. ErgoKnowledge provides interactive ergonomics training.

### LifeGuard

LifeGuard—a full-featured package available for Mac, DOS, and Windows—includes exercises for eyes and major muscle groups pertinent to computing. LifeGuard also provides basic workstation setup and posture diagrams. Its reminders are customizable—and

*Software functions as part of an overall safe-computing plan.*

■ ■ ■

**Break your computer's spell.**

■ ■ ■

**Related chapters:**

- Stretching and Exercise
- Schedules
- Eyestrain
- Stress

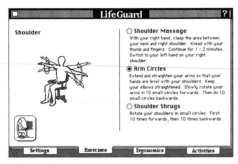

*LifeGuard*

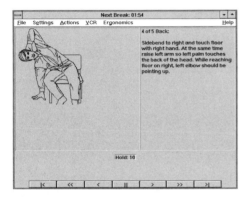

*Exercise Break*

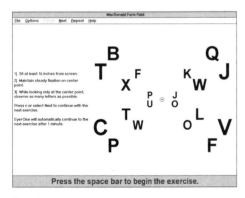

*Eyercise*

can include voice on the Mac. You determine what alternate activities LifeGuard suggests during its break prompts. LifeGuard signals you when you've exceeded your time limit of uninterrupted keyboard work—a valuable feature—but it does not flag excess keystroke intensity. $79.95 from Visionary Software. (503) 246-6200.

## Exercise Break

Exercise Break—an inexpensive package available for Mac, DOS, and Windows—contains a series of 10 exercises for the major areas of the body affected by computer use, except the eyes. Its unique Type-Watch feature records and graphically displays keyboard activity, and can switch you into Exercise Break when you exceed your predetermined keystroke intensity while in another application. Exercise Break can also be triggered by timed interval. The package includes a basic workstation chart and repetitive strain injury checklist. You can customize sets of exercises. $29.95 from Hopkins Technology. (612) 931-9376.

## Eyercise

Eyercise for Windows and OS/2 includes 19 stretches and four eye exercises. It is triggered manually or by time or interval. A triggering option beeps at you when the program is ready to run, then the exercises begin only if you stop typing for 10 seconds. Eyercise allows you to easily and extensively configure the number and duration of exercises displayed. The Eyercise package (which includes a copy of the book *Computers and Visual Stress*) is available from RAN Enterprises for $69.95. (800) 451-4487.

## User-Friendly Exercises

This solid, integrated program—available for DOS, Windows, and Mac—allows the user to choose between various exercise series, principally for the hand, wrist, back, and eye. User-Friendly Exercises' animation uses photographs, so are easy to accurately follow. The program also contains ergonomic hints and allows you to construct customized exercise series. It is triggered by timed interval. $59.95. Technically Innovative Computer Accessories distributes it through PM Ware. (800) 845-4843.

## Vision Aerobics

Vision Aerobics—available for Windows only—focuses just on the eyes. This sophisticated package contains three parts that work together as an eye-strain-reduction regimen. An arcade-style game strengthens and tones eye-movement muscles. Following geometric figures as they separate (while you wear the supplied 3-D glasses) improves depth perception. A relaxation exercise reduces overall stress. The developer claims that following the program relieves eyestrain and significantly improves visual performance. $99.00 from Vision Aerobics. (800) 445-7899.

## Take Five

Take Five, available on CD-ROM for the Mac only, takes a visual approach to computer health by providing QuickTime movies to help the user stretch and relax. Take Five also includes imagery and music intended to aid the viewer in solving problems at work. The most visually sophisticated of the computer health software packages, Take Five is user-triggered only. A Windows version was due in late 1993. $49.95 from The Voyager Company. (310) 451-1383.

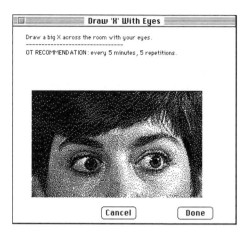

*User-Friendly Exercises*

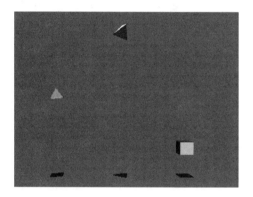

*Vision Aerobics*

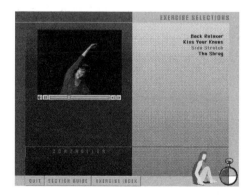

*Take Five*

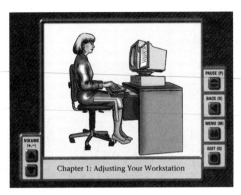

*ErgoKnowledge*

## Software Sense

Be satisfied with your selection and use of computer-health software.

**Choose it.** Evaluate different program strengths in the light of your needs. Take the program for a test drive, and don't be afraid to return it if it doesn't satisfy you.

**Use it.** All of these packages allow you to override their prompts; they'd drive you crazy if they didn't. But ignoring them can quickly become a habit. Don't let it.

**Don't abuse it.** Software is at best only part of the solution. To be effective, it must be part of an overall safe-computing strategy.

### ErgoKnowledge

ErgoKnowledge, an interactive computer-ergonomics training program for Windows and the Macintosh, trains users with a series of multimedia instructional steps. Periodic miniquizzes ensure proper learning (an incorrect answer prompts the program to review the missed material). ErgoKnowledge contains an attractive interface, talking-head narrators, and animated illustrations. It works over some networking systems. Priced on a usage basis ($395 for 10 users) from Visionary Software. (503) 246-6200.

## Do It Yourself

You can knock together some less sophisticated aid with inexpensive utility programs, one of which you may already have.

### Typing Shortcuts

Many applications (WordPerfect is just one example) have programmable macros for commonly used groups of words. Or utilities like sWord, Magic Typist, QuickKeys, WordWriter, and ProKey will enter a text string when you type a triggering keystroke combination. If you find yourself repeatedly typing the same long passages, consider checking out one of these programs to keep your keystroke count down.

### Alarms

Many macro and scheduling programs can be set up to trigger visual or aural alarms on a recurring basis. You can use different alarms to remind you to refocus, stretch, or take a break.

# Getting Medical Help

**23**

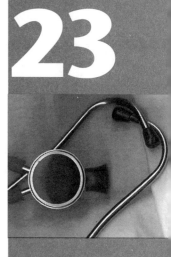

## Finding the Right Care for CTD Problems

"How do you find the right doctor?" No other question can invoke as much dismay in a chronic sufferer of a cumulative trauma disorder (CTD). Many people with computer-related CTDs have to grope their way through the medical system—often being incorrectly or inadequately diagnosed and treated—before they find someone who can give them the proper care. Many others are still looking.

This chapter describes how to find doctors for CTD problems. See **Neck and Back Pain** and **Shoulders to Hands** for more on CTD problems, and see **Glasses and Contact Lenses** and **Stress** for medical help in those areas.

### Get Help Early

If you think you have a CTD, have it checked out immediately by as good a doctor as you can find. CTD sufferers agree that putting effort into that search pays substantial benefits. The process can be daunting; you must become your own health advocate to ensure you're receiving the best care.

This chapter is intended to improve your odds. It's a compendium of information to help you find a doctor and conduct yourself in a way that increases your chances of receiving correct diagnosis and treatment.

Doctors experienced in workplace CTDs are more likely give you the best care; doctors in certain specialties are more likely to have that experience. You can narrow your search and then both question the doctor and assess the initial examination to determine if he or she is right for you. And you can prepare for the examination to help the doctor do a better job.

### Which Specialties?

A doctor with workplace CTD experience can specialize in a number of different areas. Here's a rundown.

*The wrong doctor might make things worse.*

■ ■ ■

**Few family practitioners are experienced enough in this small realm of disorders**

■ ■ ■

**Related chapters:**

- Shoulders to Hands
- Back and Neck Pain
- Changing the Workplace
- Where Else to Turn

**Occupational medicine specialists.** Occupational medicine specialists are trained to make a connection between an injury and the workplace. But some of these doctors work principally in areas like toxicology, and so may not be experienced with CTDs. Those that are board-certified in occupational medicine have had training in CTD-related injuries, and so are more likely to know what is wrong with you—as are those with physical or orthopedic medicine experience. Look for an occupational medicine specialist with particular interest in treating CTDs. When in doubt, ask about experience, training, and certification.

**Physical medicine specialists.** Physical medicine specialists are experts in the rehabilitative aspects of medicine; they are well versed in soft-tissue musculoskeletal problems. This specialty may be your best bet if you can't find an occupational medicine specialist with an interest in CTDs. Board certification in physical medicine is highly desirable.

**Orthopedic surgery specialists.** Some orthopedic surgery specialists may be appropriate—if you find the right one. Orthopedic surgery specialists are more apt to advise a significant course of nonsurgical treatment than are other types of surgeons. If you have hand or wrist pain, make sure the orthopedist treats hand injuries, which is a subspecialty of orthopedics. Also, many orthopedists will not refer to hand clinics or to physical therapy. If your orthopedist gives primarily surgical treatment, you might want to try a doctor who will take less invasive measures first. Although there are a few doctors who claim a specialty in orthopedic medicine, there are no boards in this specialty.

> ■ ■ ■
> **You must be your own health advocate.**
> ■ ■ ■

**Family practitioners, general practitioners, and internists.** Few family practitioners, general practitioners, and internists possess much experience in this small realm of disorders. It is not uncommon for less experienced doctors to make diagnoses of carpal tunnel syndrome and recommend splints or surgery when carpal tunnel syndrome is not the real problem. If you get such a recommendation and if your doctor doesn't ask questions about your work, then think about moving on. But if a family practitioner is your only option, go to her; a good family practitioner should refer you to the right specialist.

**Experienced professionals**. Other health care professionals—physical therapists, occupational therpists, recreational therapists, some specialty nurses, and some specialty psychologists, to name a few—may also be very experienced with CTDs, and be able to provide opinions, refer, or provide treatment with a doctor's orders. Knowledge and experience is the key. And some sufferers have found help from practitioners of other schools of health care, including chiropractors, acupuncturists, and massage therapists.

## Which Doctors?

Now that you know the most likely specialties, how do you narrow your search? First get recommendations. If you can't, investigate the appropriate hospitals and clinics in your area. Before proceeding farther, you may wish to check a doctor's credentials and see if she has had competency problems.

**Get recommendations.** Your goal is straightforward: find a doctor who has successfully treated conditions similar to yours. Make a list of as many CTD sufferers as you can; ask in your office, network, query your friends. Then ask each if she has found a good doctor. The emphatic affirmatives are worth following up. In a few geographical areas there are support groups and agencies that keep names of knowledgeable workplace-CTD physicians.

**Hospitals and clinics.** If you don't get a strong recommendation, you're on your own; start with the Yellow Pages. Many hospitals have occupational and physical medicine clinics; teaching hospitals associated with universities often have experienced and interested doctors who are versed in the latest procedures. You might also find a good doctor at a sports medicine clinic. Once you find a clinic, call and ask for the doctor who handles the most cases involving workplace CTDs. If the front desk can't help, ask to speak with a nurse. See *Resources*, pages 117–118, for organizations that might help you locate a clinic or physician.

**Check competence.** There's no way to determine definitively whether a doctor is competent. You can check out their credentials, however, and determine whether they've been disciplined by a state medical disciplinary board. See *Resources*, pages 117–118.

## Making the Choice

You can get a good idea as to whether a doctor has the right experience and attitude for treating your condition by questioning the doctor and appraising how well the doctor listens to and examines you. If you are not satisfied, don't be afraid to seek help elsewhere.

### Question Your Doctor
You can phone the doctor and ask the following questions as a preliminary screening method. If you cannot talk to the doctor within a few days, you may want to try someone else. How the

doctor answers your questions is just as important as what she says; you want a doctor concerned with you and your problem.

**What kinds of treatment do you offer for cumulative trauma disorders?** By the way the doctor answers, you can get an idea if she is primarily surgical or nonsurgical. You'll probably want to try nonsurgical treatment before resorting to surgery.

**Do you often suggest workplace intervention?** You want a doctor who considers the workplace in her diagnoses and is willing to suggest changes in your workplace.

**How many work-related CTD cases do you treat?** Someone in a specialty CTD clinic may see four people a day with these kinds of problems; a hand surgeon probably sees more than that.

**Do you believe that cumulative trauma disorders exist and are related to work?** Some doctors don't believe CTDs exist, but may not give you an honest answer. Accept a cautious answer—it's justified—but be leery of a hostile or evasive one.

**Do you handle Workers' Compensation cases?** If you are covered by Workers' Compensation, you need a doctor who will accept such cases. Many doctors find the paperwork and fee structure onerous.

### Get a Good Examination

If the doctor doesn't get a complete picture on the initial evaluation, she probably never will. You can improve your chances of an accurate diagnosis and a satisfying office visit with a few easy steps.

**Know your symptoms.** Do some homework—precisely determine and write down what feels or looks wrong. When did it start? How has it changed? What aggravates your pain? Can you reproduce the symptoms by putting your body in certain positions? For example, you might put your neck back or to the side, or lay down, depressing one shoulder to put traction on a neck nerve, which might produce pain—pointing to a cervical or thoracic problem. Be specific and thorough. You can interest a doctor in your case and make her job easier through a little effort.

**Describe your job**. How long do you sit at the computer, making repetitive motions? Do you assume awkward positions? Are you under deadline pressures or other psychosocial stress? Have any of your co-workers been diagnosed with CTDs? Is your workstation ergonomically sound? Many doctors familiar with computer injury realize that intervention in the workplace can aid in recovery.

**Take a friend or relative.** This isn't for everybody, but many people benefit from taking a friend or relative to the initial examination. Besides providing moral support, a friend can make sure you ask all your questions. Another set of ears and someone to discuss the interview with can be especially helpful; patients often don't remember important remarks the doctor makes during the examination.

**Take notes.** It's hard to remember everything that occurs during an interview and examination. Take notes so you can review the examination at your leisure.

**Expect an adequate examination.** The doctor needs to devote enough time to make an adequate examination and establish a relationship with you. If you don't feel like the doctor has examined you or taken a good history, you might as well give up there. On the first visit you should be asked questions similar to the following.

- How did it start?
- What makes it worse?
- What makes it better?
- What things at work aggravate it?
- What things outside of work aggravate it?

The doctor should make a complete exploration of all your symptoms. A thorough exam from the neck down is essential for proper diagnosis. If your doctor doesn't look at and feel the neck and shoulder region, you should demand it. During the examination, feel free to ask questions and make sure you understand the answers. If something is unclear, ask, ask, and ask again. Chronic CTD sufferers counsel you should be wary if you are only medicated and sent back to work, or if the doctor says, "It will go away in a couple of weeks; just wear these splints."

## Resources

A vast array of resources is available to help you find the right health care. See **Where Else to Turn** for additional descriptions and contact information.

## Educate Yourself

If you know what your condition is, understanding the diagnosis and treatment methods can help you be your own health care advocate. You can start with the public library, but for more recent (and more technical) information, try other sources. (Note: you may want to arm yourself with a medical dictionary first.)

### Medical Library
To find a medical library, call a regional office of the National Network of Libraries of Medicine (see **Where Else To Turn**). The regional office will direct you to the most appropriate medical library in your area.

### Medline
Medline, a database of articles and abstracts from over 3,600 medical journals, is available at many medical and university libraries. Increasing numbers of public libraries also have access to Medline. You may have to pay for your search.

**Finding a health care professional.** These organizations may be able to suggest clinics or physicians in your area that are experienced in treating workplace CTDs.

- American Academy of Physical Medicine & Rehabilitation. (312) 922-9366. Will supply names of physical medicine specialists in your area.

- American Occupational Medical Association (AOMA). (708) 228-6850. Will supply names of occupational medicine specialists in your area. Contact Public Relations or Education.

- Office Technology Education Project. (617) 776-2777. Located in Massachusetts.

- Committees for Occupational Safety and Health (COSHs) and affiliated organizations. Found in most states. See **Where Else to Turn**.

- RSINetwork. Support groups located primarily in the San Francisco Bay Area. Organization's newsletter is available through some on-line resources. See **Where Else to Turn** for specific subscription information.

**Checking competence.** These organizations may help you research a particular doctor's competence.

- American Board of Medical Specialties (ABMS) certification line. (800) 776-2378. This nonprofit organization provides at no charge information about doctors who are board-certified in a specialty, including the date that they were certified and for what specialties.

- Public Citizen Health Research Group. (202) 833-3000. Publishes list of doctors who have been disciplined by state boards. You can order the chapter for your state for about $10.

**Doctor-patient relations.** These two books provide tips and tricks for maximizing the care you receive from a physician.

- *Get Well, Stay Well: The Successful Patient's Handbook*, Barry Gordon, M.D. (New York: Dembner Books, 1988). A blunt yet revealing aid for dealing with doctors and the medical system. Particularly insightful in the preparations you can make that help the doctor do the best job.

- *Smart Questions to Ask Your Doctor*, Dorothy Leeds (New York: Harper Paperbacks, 1992). Useful compendium of questions to ask doctors to improve your chances of receiving the best care.

# Changing the Workplace

## Two Approaches to a Healthy Worksite

Why don't all businesses practice safe computing? Introducing ergonomic principles to the office has been shown to increase productivity while decreasing health-care costs, absenteeism, and turnover. Morale generally improves because most employees view an ergonomics program as an indication that their company is interested in their welfare. Besides, some employees with computer-related cumulative trauma disorders (CTDs) have recently begun to sue their employers—and some have won. Yet many companies still need to be convinced that this change is in their best interests. In the office, change does not often come easily.

For those managers who need no convincing, an ergonomics program can be created to make the organization ergonomically self-sufficient. Or, effective change can come from the bottom up, if you know how.

## The Perfect Working Environment

The perfect working environment—where the risks of injury are reduced to their minimum—is an ideal realized by no company. In order to reduce job injuries, a number of businesses have asked the National Institute for Occupational Safety and Health (NIOSH) to investigate the sources of work-related musculoskeletal disorders and recommend solutions. Although all of NIOSH's recommendations cannot be applied to every company or situation, they are useful as signposts to the elusive risk-free workplace.

**Breaks.** Make sure that employees take frequent breaks away from their workstations. Consider using software-activated break alerts. See **Schedules** and **Software**.

**Reduce psychological stress.** Give employees a voice in decision-making. Encourage their involvement in their job design. Inform them of how to advance in company. Let them know what to expect in the company's future. Support policies of job diversity and job security. See **Stress**.

*Good ergonomics increases productivity.*

■ ■ ■

**Change can come from the bottom or the top.**

■ ■ ■

## Related chapters:

- Schedules
- Software
- Stress
- Where Else to Turn

# Is Everyone Involved?

*In the ideal office, safety awareness stretches throughout the hierarchy of the organization.*

**Management.** *Is management actively promoting ergonomic awareness? Does management seek out potential injury advice from employees?*

**Supervisors.** *Are supervisors rewarded on just the performance of their group, or also on low injury rates among their employees?*

**Employees.** *Are employees actively involved in trying to improve ergonomics—and in promoting the advantages to both workers and employers that can result? Do employees' job evaluations consider if they taking their rest breaks and adhering to safety principles?*

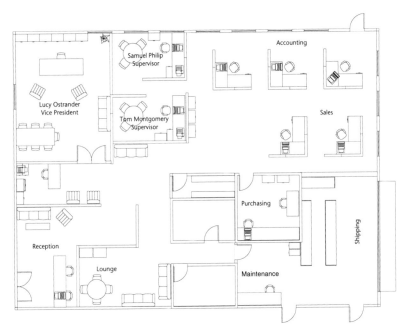

**Purchasing.** *Does purchasing choose products based on what's cheapest, or on what really works the best? Does purchasing systematically evaluate available products?*

**Maintenance.** *Does equipment work correctly? Are manufacturers' warranties being utilized or wasted?*

**Reduce keystrokes.** Modify deadline orientation. Ensure adequate personnel for jobs demanding intense keyboarding. Rotate jobs. See if the keyboard-intensive tasks can be replaced with another entry method (like using optical character recognition). Eliminate typing quotas; focus on typists reducing errors instead.

**Physical environment.** Ensure that the workplace is ergonomically sound. Good ergonomic furniture and equipment increases productivity. See **The Chair, The Desk, Keyboards and Mice,** and **The Perfect Workstation**.

**Training.** Make sure the employees have been trained in sound ergonomic principles and in their application to each worker's particular equipment. See *Resources*, page 125, for training materials.

**Encourage a safety-first environment.** Make sure workers who suspect they are injured receive immediate medical evaluation without fear of reprisal. Make someone responsible for ergonomic issues. Periodically review site safety.

## From the Top Down

Management that desires a safe workplace typically employs an ergonomics consultant (see *Finding an Ergonomist* at right) who tries to make their client ergonomically self-sufficient. A typical ergonomics program contains most of the following elements.

### Planning

In the planning stage, the structure to institute change is formed, the ergonomic requirements of the worksite are evaluated, and an overall plan is developed.

**Management support.** Management supports an ergonomics program by providing the resources and structure to help identify and abate ergonomic hazards. Management also communicates their support for the program to all employees.

**Ergonomics committee.** An ergonomics committee is formed that involves different departments and various levels of management; diversity is an asset. The committee is trained in ergonomic principles and becomes responsible for ergonomic change throughout the organization.

**Worksite evaluation.** The committee evaluates the workplace, including the physical setup, people, tasks, organizational structure, and reward policies. Medical and insurance records are often reviewed to pinpoint problems. Employees are encouraged to make complaints or suggestions; employees are an invaluable source of hazard information.

**Written plan.** The committee formulates a long-term plan, and ensures that proper timetables and checks are instituted so that it will move forward. Money and time are budgeted for the program.

## Finding an Ergonomist

The proliferation of office injuries has been accompanied by an increase in "ergonomics consultants," some of whom may not have the necessary qualifications to do a good job. The Human Factors and Ergonomics Society publishes a directory of human factors and ergonomics consultants. The right ergonomics consultant should meet the following criteria.

- Wants to develop the client's internal expertise in ergonomics.

- Doesn't have a single fixed solution.

- Addresses the psychosocial area, not just physical issues.

- Doesn't necessarily want to sell you equipment.

- Proposes a long-range plan, not cheap, quick fixes.

- Gives you a detailed bid that lists all services to be provided.

The consultant you choose should have the following experience.

- Formal training in ergonomics or in a closely related field such as industrial psychology.

- At least five years of work experience in the field.

Be sure to ask for and check out references.

## Free Hazards Consultation

The US Department of Labor's Occupational Safety and Health Administration (OSHA) and the Canadian Workers' Compensation Boards provide free and confidential consultations and information on worksite problems and hazards Depending on the severity and type of problem, the federal or local occupational safety and health authority may send inspectors, letters, or brochures to help insure compliance with worksite safety regulations. In the US, the National Institute of Occupational Safety and Health (NIOSH) also has an 800 number for requesting information and rarely given worksite evaluations. See *Resources*, page 125, and **Where Else to Turn** for whom to call in your area.

## Implementing

Once ergonomic hazards are identified, the next step is to design measures to prevent or control them.

**Training and education.** Training allows managers, supervisors, and employees to understand ergonomic hazards. Then the whole worksite can participate actively in the protection process. Education must meet specific needs; for example, employees need real-world training in furniture adjustment, correct posture, and stretching exercises.

**Intervention.** The ergonomics committee institutes the most necessary fixes first. Medical management is introduced to reduce the risk of injury by early identification and treatment. (At this time the number of problems may actually seem to increase, because they are being identified sooner.) Often a model project is implemented first to demonstrate the efficacy of the program. There can be an advantage in going slow: the committee can make changes, see how people react, and incorporate the feedback into refinements of the program.

**Evaluation.** In most programs, there will be more improvement in some areas than others. Continuing problems are addressed. Eventually, a company-wide awareness of ergonomics should be in place.

## From the Bottom Up

Concerned that your workplace is injuring people? You've tried internal grievance procedures and your supervisor or employer doesn't seem to be listening? As a worker, you have three courses of action.

**Contact governmental authorities.** In the US, contact the regional offices of OSHA or their equivalent in state government. In Canada, get in touch with the provincial or territorial Workers' Compensation Board. These agencies have the power to force companies to comply with safe work practices or will get an enforcement authority involved. If there is an immediate health-threatening hazard in the workplace, call one of the numbers listed in *Resources*, page 125, or in **Where Else to Turn**. These organizations can also provide useful information for designing and promoting workplace change.

**Use your union.** If you are in a union, you can use your union representative as a primary source of help. In the short term, your union should help fix the problem; in the long term, unions are successfully bargaining for contracts that incorporate video-display terminal safety clauses.

**Change the workplace.** If you are not in a union, seek out other workers as both allies and sources of information, then use the following strategy to implement workplace change.

## Identify Problems
Document the suspected hazards by investigating work areas, equipment, job designs, and schedules. Use ergonomic guidelines and checklists available from a number of organizations (see *Resources*, below). If you find that people are injured, make sure they seek medical assistance immediately.

> ■ ■ ■
> **Slow change can have advantages.**
> ■ ■ ■

## List Hazards and Develop Solutions
Brainstorm solutions with fellow workers. Then list the solutions in three categories.

**Immediate fixes.** The fast, no-cost, band-aid solutions that workers can do themselves, such as moving equipment or adjusting chairs.

**Midrange fixes.** Those medium-cost solutions that need employer involvement.

**Larger fixes.** These solutions will costs the employer an appreciable amount, so their implementation will probably need to be negotiated.

## Write Up Your Study
Prioritize and set realistic goals. What must you have now and what can be put off until later? Be sure to set the highest priority on help for those who are already injured. A good strategy in an initial request is to include one low-cost solution (like a copy stand) needed by many workers. This gets management involved and shows workers that they can promote change.

## Present the Study to the Employer
One possible way is through a health and safety committee. Point out that many of the changes can be simple and inexpensive. Provide evidence that ergonomic change is cost-effective and

# Americans with Disabilities Act

The Americans with Disabilities Act prevents discrimination against the disabled, including those disabled on the job—like those who have gotten carpal tunnel syndrome from keyboarding. The act requires the employer to make reasonable accommodation to keep a disabled worker on the payroll, which in most situations means employers acquire special equipment, give training, or design jobs to comply. The government has funded the Job Accommodation Network to confidentially advise companies how to deal with a particular disability case. See **Where Else to Turn** for phone numbers to call for a free consultation.

increases productivity. Your regional OSHA office or Workers' Compensation Board, a local National Safety Council office, or your company's workers' compensation insurance carrier are good places to find supporting information.

## Legal Issues

Both employers and their employees should be aware of the legal environment surrounding computer injury. Laws and regultions may vary from state to state, and some are rapidly changing.

### Workers' Compensation.

State workers' compensation systems mostly developed in the late 1800s and early 1900s to compensate injured workers for medical costs, lost wages, and rehabilitation expenses. In return for the assurance of compensation, the employee gave up the right to sue the employer for injurious working conditions. Workers' compensation laws and their implementation may vary widely between states, especially in regard to CTDs. Some states still resist compensating for CTDs, suggesting that a direct connection to the workplace has not been made.

### OSHA Regulations

In order to ensure worker safety, the federal and state governments have Occupational Safety and Health Administrations (OSHA). Up until now, OSHA has dealt with CTDs on an industry basis, most notably creating a set of ergonomic guidelines for the meat packing industry, where OSHA was responsible for identifying ergonomic risks. But recently OSHA announced its intention to speedily create an industry-wide set of ergonomics regulations that would include the computerized workplace, where the obligation of recognizing risks would shift to business.

It's impossible to predict the final form of these regulations due to the battle of special interest groups and other concerned parties that will influence the final outcome. Experts predict that regulations may be in place in early 1996. Meanwhile, one state, California, intends to have ergonomic regulations in place by the beginning of 1995.

# Resources

These resources can be useful in ensuring safe working conditions and changing the workplace. Also see **Where Else to Turn**.

**Office Technology Education Project.** (617) 776-2777. This nonprofit organization provides education services and resources to computer users about the health and job impact of technology. Their aim is to ensure that computer users enjoy the benefits promised by the new technology.

**9to5, National Association of Working Women.** (414) 274-0925. This nonprofit organization provides information on worker safety, workplace monitoring, and advocating for workers' rights.

**The Association for Repetitive Motion Syndromes**. (707) 571-3097. This nonprofit organization provides information on RSI. They accept calls 10 am to 5 pm Pacific Time only.

**COSHs and related organizations.** Committees for Occupational Safety and Health. Labor-oriented organizations that provide information on worker health, productivity, and workplace change. See **Where Else to Turn** for your region's COSH.

**NIOSH.** (800) 356-4674. In some circumstances the National Institute of Occupational Safety and Health will study worksites and make recommendations to ensure healthy working conditions.

**OSHA.** State or Federal OSHA offices can provide information and resources. Call regional OSHA office, listed in **Where Else to Turn**. Free OSHA publications: *Ergonomics Program Management Recommendations for General Industry, Handbook for Small Business,* and *Record Keeping Guidelines for Occupational Injuries and Illnesses. ErgoFacts*, OSHA's free quarterly publication on improving workplace ergonomics.

**Publications.** Human Factors and Ergonomics Society. (310) 394-1811. Publishes directory of human factors and ergonomics consultants organized geographically and available for $35 to non-members or $20 to members.

"Office Ergonomics Management Program." Pamphlet to guide management in instituting ergonomic change. Center for Office Technology. (703) 276-1174.

"ADA Technical Manual." First copy is free from a distribution center operated for the Equal Employment Opportunities Committee. (800) 669-3362.

> ■ ■ ■
> **OSHA intends to quickly enact ergonomic regulations.**
> ■ ■ ■

# 25 Where Else to Turn

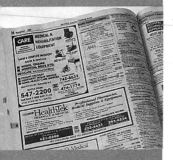

## Safe Computing Resources

**From software to medical libraries, staying healthy at the computer is up to you.**

■ ■ ■

**Let the buyer beware.**

■ ■ ■

Inside *Zap!* you can find most of what you need to stay healthy at the computer—but no book can do it all. Looking elsewhere for products, information, and expertise can be a daunting and frustrating experience, so here's some help.

We've listed resources by company or organization name; if they have one or two products for their category, it is noted after the company name. Most organizations have toll-free 800 numbers accessible throughout the United States and Canada. But we've also listed the toll number where available. The information below was accurate as of publication time, but things change; we'll keep this list updated in subsequent editions.

Where US federal and state agencies and US national organizations are listed, we have also included their Canadian counterparts where appropriate.

## Software

**Don Johnston's Developmental Equipment** (Co:Writer), PO Box 639, 1000 N. Rand Rd. Bldg. 115, Wauconda, IL 60084. (800) 999-4660 or (708) 526-2682. Fax (708) 526-4177. Word-prediction program.

**FingerTip Info** (User Friendly Exercises). Distributed by PM Ware, 346 State Place, Escondido, CA 92029. (800) 845-4843 or (619) 738-6633.

**Hopkins Technology** (Exercise Break), 421 Hazel Lane, Hopkins, MN 55343-7116. (612) 931-9376. Fax (612) 931-9377.

**RAN Enterprises** (Eyercise), 1 Woodland Park Dr., Haverhill, MA 01830. (800) 451-4487 or (508) 521-4487.

**Shareware.** Power Clicks. a $3 shareware program that activates the mouse button with a keystroke. Written by Alessandro Levi Montalcini. Available through the Internet by anonymous FTP to sumex-aim.stanford.edu and its mirrors under the path info-mac/cfg/power-clicks-102.hqx.

**Sonera Technologies** (DisplayMate), PO Box 565, Rumson, NJ 07760. (800) 932-6323 or (908) 747-6886. The most advanced diagnostic software for monitors. $149.

**the sWord**, PO Box 176, Comptche, CA 95427-0176. (707) 937-4298. Abbreviation-typing program for Mac and PC (for example, type a "u" and you get the word "you").

**Vision Aerobics** (Vision Aerobics). Distributed by Programmers' Paradise, 1163 Shrewsbury, Shrewsbury, NJ 07702. (800) 445-7899.

**Visionary Software** (LifeGuard and ErgoKnowledge), 1820 SW Vermont Suite A, Portland, OR 97219. (503) 246-6200. Computer-health training and support programs.

**Voyager Company** (Take Five), 1351 Pacific Coast Highway, Santa Monica, CA 90401. (800) 446-2001 or (310) 451-1383. CD-ROM-based set of physical and relaxation exercises.

*See also Keyboard Alternatives: Fountain Hill Systems, Inc; Hand and Arm Supports: Ergodyne; Organizations: TCO.*

## Workstation Furniture

**Agio Designs**, 1400 NW Compton Dr., Beaverton, OR 97006. (800) 688-2446 or (503) 690-1400. Mac and PC furniture and computer accessories, such as keyboard trays and lamps.

**American Ergonomics Corp**, PO Box 2848, Sausalito, CA 94966-2848. (415) 332-5635. Fax (415) 332-1806. Ergomax, unique chair with floating seat that responds to body motion.

**Amotek/Lusa Inc**, 1730 State St., Bridgeport, CT 06605. (800) 242-4777 or (203) 576-9086. Ergonomic seating and adjustable-height tables.

**Anthro Company**, 3221 NW Yeon St., Portland, OR 97210. (800) 325-3841 or (503) 241-7113. Adjustable desks and accessories.

**BackCare Corporation**, 200 South Desplaines Ave., Chicago, IL 60661. (312) 258-0888. Fax (312) 258-0090. Imports, distributes, and retails some Swedish seating and other furniture.

**BackSaver Products Company**, 53 Jeffrey Avenue, Holliston, MA 01746. (800) 251-2225 or (508) 429-5940. Chairs and body supports.

### Smart Shopper

Most software and hardware is available through distributors at a discount off suggested retail price—sometimes as much as 50 percent off. Check computer catalogs and magazines for listings for anything you're interested in; call the manufacturer if you want product literature or if you can't find a distributor.

■ ■ ■
**Remember: no one certifies ergonomic design.**
■ ■ ■

**Bevco Precision Manufacturing Co**, W227 N752 Westmound Drive, Suite. L3A, Waukesha, WI 53186. (414) 547-6990. Fax (414) 547-8225. Chairs.

**Biofit Engineered Seating**, PO Box 109, Watterville, OH 43566. (800) 597-0246 or (419) 823-1089. Chairs.

**Bodybilt Seating**, 3900 Texas Avenue South, College Station, TX 77845-5831. (800) 364-5673. Fax (409) 764-1935. Highly adjustable seating that helps body emulate a gravity-free environment.

**Charvoz-Dauphin**, 180 Passaic Avenue, Fairfield, NJ 07004. (800) 631-1186. Office seating.

**Corel Seating, Inc**, 330 Ashland Road, PO Box 1991, Mansfield, OH 44901. (800) 537-5573. Seating.

**EckAdams Company**, 347 N. Lindbergh Boulevard, St. Louis, MO 63141-7888. (800) 333-7328. Office chairs and stools.

**Ergogenic Technology Inc**, 45 Appletree Lane, Pipersville, PA 18947. (215) 766-8545. Fax (215) 766-8599. Adjustable workstations.

**Ergonomic Logic, Inc**, 205 Vista Blvd., #101, Sparks, NV 89434. (800) 527-6600 or (702) 331-6001. Fax (702) 331-9060. European-design office chairs and workstation accessories including monitor stands, articulating arm supports, and foot rests.

**Ergonomic Sciences Corp**, 2672 Bayshore Parkway, Suite 520, Mountain View, CA 94043. (415) 964-3135. Fax (800) 283-9444. Selected workstation furniture and accessories.

**Ergotron**, 3450 Yankee Dr. Suite 100, Eagan, MN 55121. (800) 888-8458 or (612) 452-8135. Workstation racks, stands, and suspension components.

**Fixtures Furniture**, 1642 Crystal, Kansas City, MO 64126. (800) 821-3500 or (816) 241-4500. Fax (816) 241-4027. Wide variety of seating.

**Girsberger Office Seating**, PO Box 1476, Smithfield, NC 27577. (800) 849-0545. Variety of office seating.

**Global Industries**, 17 West Stow Road, Marlton, NJ 08053. (800) 220-1900. Desks and chairs.

**Grahl Industries, Inc,** One Grahl Drive, PO Box 345, Coldwater, MI 49036. (517) 279-8011. Ergonomic, adjustable chairs.

**Hag**, 108 Landmark Dr., Greensboro, NC 27409. (800) 334-4839 or (919) 668-9541. Office chairs.

**Hamilton Sorter Co, Inc,** PO Box 18008, Fairfield, OH 45018-0008. (800) 543-1605 or (513) 870-4400. Freestanding desks, workstations, and mailroom furniture.

**Haworth, Inc,** One Haworth Center, Holland, MI 49423. (800) 344-2600 or (616) 393-3000. Complete office systems.

**Herman Miller, Inc,** 855 E. Main St., Zeeland, MI 49464. (616) 772-3300. Furniture, workstations.

**ISE**, 25300 Northline Road, Taylor, MI 48180. West (800) 835-3595, Central (800) 982-4702, East (800) 272-2950, Canada (800) 463-7731. Workstations, chairs, and ergonomic consultation.

**The Knoll Group**, 655 Madison Ave., New York, NY 10021. (212) 207-2200. Office systems and high-end home furnishings.

**Marvel Group, Inc,** 3843 West 43rd St., Chicago, IL 60632. (800) 621-8846. Fax (800) 237-0358. Office furniture and seating.

**Metier**, PO Box 4120, Pineville, LA 71361-4120. (318) 640-8170. Fax (318) 640-8184. Sit-stand workstations.

**MicroCentre**, Continental Engineering Group, Inc, 5300 North Irwindale Ave. Irwindale, CA 91706. (800) 966-5511 or (818) 338-0870. Workstations.

**Miller Desk Co.**, Drawer HP-11, High Point, NC 27261. (800) 438-4324. Office seating.

**Navigator Systems/Dean Santner Design**, 4210 Holden Street, PO Box 88185, Emeryville, CA 94662. (415) 653-9385 or (415) 653-9300. Workstation desks designed by master woodworker.

**Neutral Posture**, 2301 Fountain Avenue, Bryan, TX 77801. (409) 822-5080. Fax (409) 775-1963. Adjustable seating.

**Nova Office Furniture, Inc,** 421 W. Industrial Avenue, Effington, IL 62401. (217) 342-7070. Fax (217) 342-7006. Monitor-below-work surface computer furniture. Adjustable height keyboard trays. Offers booklet, *VDT Workstation Handbook*, a particularly informative and well-written source on office-ergonomics.

**Paralax**, 2550 W. Midway Blvd., Broomfield, CO 80020. (800) 972-7259. Desks and workstations.

**ScanCo**, PO Box 3217, Redmond, WA 98073-3217. (800) 722-6263 or (206) 481-5434. Computer tables and other furniture.

**SIS Human Factor Technologies, Inc,** 55 Harvey Road, Londonerry, NH 03053. (603) 432-4495. Height adjustable computer furniture, wrist and foot rests, accessories.

**Southern Technical Associates**, 11498 Raleigh Lagrange Rd., Eads, TN 38028. (901) 853-0023. Security desk.

**Steelcase, Inc,** Grand Rapids, MI 49501. (616) 247-2710. Office furniture, accessories, and lighting equipment including modular workstations and fully adjustable chairs and desks.

**VuRyte, Inc,** 1530 South SW Loop 323, Suite 111, Tyler, TX 75701. (800) 678-2629 or (903) 593-4666. Workstations and monitor pedestals; transparent, adjustable document holders.

*See also Hand and Arm Supports: MicroComputer Accessories.*

## Alternative Input

**Apple Computer, Inc,** 1 Infinite Loop, Cupertino, CA 95014. (408) 996-1010. PlainTalk voice-recognition software works on most Macintosh systems and is bundled with Power Macintoshes, allows voice control of some system functions. No training of system is required, although some controls are available. Third parties are now releasing additional support to allow dictation and other control.

**Articulate Systems**, 600 West Cummings Park, Suite 4500, Woburn, MA 01801. (617) 935-5656. Fax (617) 935-0490. Voice-recognition products, including hardware—such as Voice Navigator II, a complete voice input system—and software like Power-Secretary, a dictation program designed by Dragon Systems (see listing below).

**Command Corp., Inc** (IN3), 3761 Venture Drive, Duluth, GA 30136. (404) 813-8030. Fax (404) 813-0113. IN3 Voice Command lets users replace repetitive mouse and keyboard motions with voice macros. Requires no proprietary hardware. Platforms: PCs with Windows 3.1, Sun.

**Dragon Systems, Inc** (DragonDictate-30K), 320 Nevada Street, Newton, MA 02160. (800) 825-5897 or (617) 965-5200. Fax (617) 527-0372. Sophisticated speech-recognition software.

**IBM Corporation** (Personal Dictation System), (800) 825-5263. Speech-recognition systems for PCs.

**Kurzweil Applied Intelligence, Inc** (Voice), 411 Waverly Oaks Road, Waltham, MA 02154. (800) 380-1234. Fax (617) 893-6525. Voice-recognition system for Windows.

**Madenta**, 9411A-20 Avenue, Edmonton, Alberta T6N 1E5 Canada. (800) 661-8406 or (403) 450-8926. Fax (403) 428-5376. AppleLink:

Madenta. Software for disabled people including: voice recognition, typing without the use of hands, using a computer with limited body motion.

## Mouse Alternatives

**Kraft Systems**, 450 W. California Ave., Vista, CA 92083. (619) 724-7146. Fax (619) 941-1770. Trackball and footpedal combination, joysticks.

**Logitech, Inc** (MouseMan), 6505 Kaiser Dr., Fremont, CA 94555. (800) 231-7717 or (510) 795-8100. Large mouse with programmable buttons.

**MicroTouch Systems, Inc** (UnMouse), 300 Griffin Park, Methuen, MA 01844. (508) 694-9900. Fax (508) 659-9100. Touch tablet that replaces mouse. Can be configured so that screen cursor tracks when you move your finger on tablet, or the tablet can act as a programmable keypad.

*See also Screen Accessories: Kensington, Keyboard Alternatives: Microsoft.*

## Keyboard Alternatives

**Applied Learning Corp.** (Maltron), Box 686, King of Prussia, PA 19406. (215) 688-6866. Oldest alternative layout design. QWERTY (or other arrangement of keys) set in two separate contoured "dishes." Compatible with PC and Mac.

**ErgoLogic Enterprises, Inc**, 47000 Warm Springs Blvd., Unit 430, Fremont, CA 94539-7467. (800) 665-9929. Identical to Key Tronics FlexPro.

**ErgonomiXX, Inc** (MyKey Ergonomic Keyboard), 525-K East Market St., Box 295, Leesburg, VA 22075. (703) 771-1047. Fax (703) 771-1137. CompuServe: 75050, 3323. Contoured shape using QWERTY layout. Mouse and function keys in keypad at left. Not adjustable, but relatively inexpensive. Compatible with PC.

**Fountain Hill Systems, Inc** (FH-101), 15022 N. 75th Street, Miami Lakes, FL 33014. (602) 596-8633. Fax (602) 948-1925. V-shaped keyboard that comes with exercise software.

**Handykey Corporation** (Twiddler), 141 Mount Sinai Ave., Mount Sinai, NY 11766. (800) 638-2352 or (516) 474-4405. Relatively inexpensive 12-key chord keyboard that straps into hand. Also incorporates mouse pointing device. Compatible with PC.

**Health Care Keyboard Systems** (Comfort Keyboard), N82 W15340 Appleton Avenue, Menomonee Falls, WI 53051. (414) 253-6333. Fax (414) 253-6330. Highly adjustable, three-way-split keyboard. Compatible with PC, Mac, Sun, others.

**Industrial Innovations, Inc** (DataHand), 10789 North 90th St. Suite 201, Scottsdale, AZ 85260. (602) 860-8584. Unusual five-finger keyboard in which fingers rest in molded cups that pick up five different directions of movement. Compatible with PC and Mac.

**Infogrip, Inc** (Bat), 812 North Blvd., Baton Rouge, LA 70802. (800) 397-0921 or (504) 336-0033. Seven-key chording keyboard. Operates in one hand although for faster input, another unit can be operated simultaneously with the other hand. Compatible with PC and Mac.

**InHand Development Group** (DataEgg), (916) 983-2249. One-handed notetaking, chord-key device with seven buttons (three for thumb, one for each remaining fingers); chording with these buttons can generate all keyboard and control characters. Shipping late 1994.

**Key Tronic Corporation** (FlexPro), PO Box 14687, Spokane, WA 99214-0687. (509) 928-8000. Fax (509) 927-5224. Adjustable split keyboard. *See also* ErgoLogic

**Kinesis** (Kinesis Ergonomic Keyboard), 915 118th Avenue SE, Bellevue, WA 98005-3855. (206) 455-9220. QWERTY layout with keys located in separate, dished positions, a design the manufacturer claims will reduce strain on the hands and wrists. Compatible with PC and Mac.

**Lexmark International, Inc** (Select-Ease), 740 New Circle Rd NW, Lexington, KY 40511-1876. (800) 438-2468. Relatively inexpensive split keyboard for PCs.

**Marquardt Switches, Inc** (MiniErgo), 2711 Route 20 East, Cazenovia, NY 13035. (800) 282-3746. Fax (315) 655-8042. Inexpensive divided keyboard of European manufacture. Keypad that can be positioned on either side also available. Compatible with PC.

**Microsoft Corporation** (Natural Keyboard), One Microsoft Way, Redmond, WA 98052-6399. (206) 882-8080. Contoured design. PC-compatible only. Also, a PC-compatible contoured mouse.

**Somers Engineering** (EK1), 3424 Vicker Way, Palmdale, CA 93551. (805) 273-1609. Standard-looking keyboard with alphanumeric keys set out in a grid instead of staggered. Compatible with PC and Mac.

**Vatell Corporation** (AccuKey), PO Box 66, Christianberg, VA 24073. (703) 961-3576. Fax (703) 953-3010. Molded eight-key keyboard, designed to rest in lap, in which all characters are entered as two-fingered chords, using one finger on each hand. Compatible with PC, Mac, Sun, and other platforms.

**Workplace Designs, Inc,** 301-311 S. Main Street, Stillwater, MN 55082. (715) 549-5922. Split keyboard mounted on chair arms.

## EMR Shields

**Get Safe! Inc** (ELF Armor), PO Box 139, Fairfield, IA 52556. (515) 472-5551. Manufactures and installs ELF Armor, an alloy cylinder mounted over the monitor's deflection coil that reduces magnetic field emissions.

**NoRad Corporation**, 1160 E. Sandhill Ave., Carson, CA 90746. (310) 395-0800. Produces devices to reduce magnetic and electric fields. A new product, the JitterBox, is designed to eliminate monitor image jitter and distortion from magnetic-field interference.

*See also Organizations: Safety First Association.*

## Screen Accessories

**American Optical** (Truevision Technica Lens), (508) 765-9711. Manufactures a prescription-only spectacle lens designed for computer users.

**Curtis Manufacturing Co.** (MVP Mouse), 30 Fitzgerald Drive, Jaffrey, New Hampshire 03452. (603) 532-4123. Copy stands, wrist rests, glare filters, monitor stands, and other accessories.

**Kensington Microware**, 2855 Campus Drive, San Mateo, CA 94403. (415) 572-2700 or (800) 535-4242. Computer accessories: stands, mice, protection devices, and carrying cases.

**Less Gauss**, PO Box 5006, Rhinebeck, NY 12572. (800) 872-1051 or (914) 876-5432. Manufactures glare filters (optical glass, quartz-fused finish) in three tints; magnifier that is suspended from monitor top which can be slid forward and back. Also mouse supports and wrist rests.

**Optical Coating Laboratory, Inc,** Glare/Guard Division, 2789 Northpoint Parkway, Santa Rosa, CA 95407-7397. (800) 545-6254. Glass glare shields from a leading optical-coating company.

**Optical Devices, Inc,** 805 Via Alondra, Camarillo, CA 93012. (805) 987-8801. Fax (805) 388-1123. Circular polarizing and non-polarizing glare filters.

**Polaroid Corp.**, 1 Upland Rd., N2-1K, Norwood, MA 02062. (800) 225-2770. Fax (617) 446-4600. Offers a range of circular polarizing glare filters. Most are also antistatic.

**Reach Industries**, 5776 Nakat Way, Birch Bay, WA 98230. (800) 663-8764. Fax (206) 371-7226. Antistatic glare filter; 30-day trial.

**The Rosenblum Company, Inc** (Made in the Shade), 412 Country Club Dr., San Francisco, CA 94132-1112. (415) 665-2020. Anti-glare, antistatic computer visor attaches to monitor with Velcro.

**Soft/View Computer Products**, 2 Fox Point Center, Suite 100, 6 Denny Road, Wilmington, DE 19809. (302) 762-9229. Fax (302) 762-9210. Established maker of popular glass glare shields. Also markets wrist and foot rests and other accessories.

*See also Furniture: VuRyte, Inc.*

## Hand and Arm Supports

**Able Table Co.** (Able Table), 227 Fern St., Santa Cruz, CA 95060. (408) 425-5767. The Able Table portable table (about the size of a breakfast-in-bed tray) supports reading material or laptop computer in almost any position.

**Aqua-Cel Corp.** (Aqua-Cel Pain Relief Pads), PO Box 26827, Santa Anna, CA 92799. (714) 962-2776. Various sizes of gel-filled pads for heating or cooling body therapy.

**Custom Comfort Ergonomics**, 4102 E. 7th St. Suite 260, Long Beach, CA 90804. (800) 488-3746 or (310) 438-8951. Fax (310) 434-3894. Pillows to hold keyboard or laptop on your lap; footrest with foot-massage feature.

**Ergodyne**, 1410 Energy Park Drive, St. Paul, MN 55108. (800) 225-8238. Fax (612) 642-1882. Hand, arm, back, and foot supports. Video-based training programs. Stretching software.

**ErgoFlex** (DataArms), 4917 Chippewa Dr., Larkspur, CO 80118. (800) 788-2810 or (303) 681-2221. Designed to take the strain off shoulders and neck. Articulating forearm support device said to benefit the shoulders and neck. Plus, a variety of accessories and furniture intended to benefit health at the computer.

**Ergonomic Design Inc,** 10650 Irma Drive, #33, Northglenn, CO 80233. (800) 645-5122 or (303) 452-8006. Fax (303) 452-2296. Wrist and foot rests, keyboard supports, document holders.

**Fox Bay Industries, Inc,** 4150 "B" Place N. W., Auburn, WA 98001. (800) 874-8527. Wrist supports, foot, and lumbar supports. Other accessories including drawer slides.

**LB Innovators, Inc,** 2524 Main Street, Suite H, Chula Vista, CA 91911. (800) 754-2383 or (708) 397-9180. Fax (619) 423-2383. Wrist and foot rests, glare filters, notebook travel case, other accessories.

**Microcomputer Accessories** (The Wrist Reminder and The Wrist Trolley), 9920 LaCienega Blvd. 12th floor, Inglewood, CA 90302. (800) 521-8270 or (310) 645-9400. Reminder is a strap-on wrist brace. Trolley is a pair of wrist support pads that glide along a track as you move your hands from side to side while typing. Also furniture.

**MouseMitt International**, 75 Green Valley Road, Scotts Valley, CA 95066. (408) 335-9599. Fax (408) 335-9598. Two kinds of padded, fingerless gloves.

**Myonetics** (Arm), PO Box 373099, Satellite Beach, FL 32937-1099. (407) 779-9876. Fax (407) 779-9877. Unique, fully articulating forearm supports that extend from base under keyboard and mouse.

**Padware, Inc,** 166 Forbes Road, Braintree, MA 02814. (800) 577-2698. Wrist rests, foot rests, back rest, mouse cover, and other accessories.

**Patternworks, Inc** (MediLycra), PO Box 1690, Poughkeepsie, NY 12601. (800) 438-5464 or (914) 462-8000. They make a Lycra glove treated with a patented process that traps heat in the hands and acts as a support. The company claims that people can do a repetitive activity longer without hands being strained.

**ShadowTech International, Inc** (Mouseshadow), 1104 Northwest 73rd Street, Lawton, OK 73505. (800) 392-1402 or (405) 536-7108. Wrist-elevation device that moves with your mouse.

**Silicon Sports**, 324 High Street, Palo Alto, CA 94301. (800) 243-2972 or (415) 327-7900. Fax (415) 327-7962. Screen-saver software, mouse pads, wrist rests, and integrated supports for wrists, hands, and mice.

*See also Furniture: Ergonomic Logic, BackCare Corporation; Organizations: TCO; Screen Accessories: Less Gauss.*

## Telephone Headsets

**ACS Communications**, 10 Victor Square, Scotts Valley, CA 95066. (800) 995-5500. Referrals to local distributors of their products.

**GBH Distributing**, 701 West Harvard Street, Glendale, CA 91204. (800) 222-5424. Headsets, telephones, chairs, and computer accessories.

**Mr. Headset,** PO Box 350187, Grand Island, FL 32735-0187. (800) 332-8668.

**Plantronics**, Santa Cruz, CA. (800) 544-4660.

**Unex Telephone Headsets**, 27 Industrial Ave. Chelmsford, MA 01824. (800) 345-8639 or (508) 256-8222. Fax (508) 250-9055.

**Wicom**, 9851 Owensmouth Avenue, Chatsworth, CA 91311. (800) 517-5400.

## Miscellaneous Accessories

**AliMed Incorporated**, 297 High St., Dedham, MA 02026. (800) 225-2610 or (617) 329-2900. Fax (617) 329 8392. Wide range of ergonomic office, industrial, and computer supports, furniture, and supplies.

**Allegro Industries**, 6403 E. Alondra Blvd., Paramount, CA 90723. (800) 622-3530 or (310) 633-4861. Fax (310) 633-2224. Catalog of back, wrist, hand, and other body supports; mostly intended for police, fire, and medical personnel, but also have computer products.

**B&L Industries** (Deskalator), 1329 Plum St., Lincoln, NE 68502. (800) 544-5299. Fax (402) 435-4047. Inexpensive device to raise desk height.

**Bio-Lite Marketing, Inc,** 431 Seabreeze Ave., Palm Beach, FL 33480. (800) 678-8181. Bio-Lite desk light that produces flicker-free, continuous-spectrum light at the same color as early-morning sunlight; claimed will help avoid strain and fatigue.

**Equipment Direct**, PO Box 670, Yorba Linda, CA 92686. (800) 424-4410. Glare shields, wrist supports, seating, and workstations.

**Keytime**, 4516 NE 54th Street, Seattle, WA 98105-2933. (206) 324-7219. Keycap stickers for Dvorak layout. Typing instruction.

**Master Mfg. Co. Inc,** 9200 Inman Ave., Cleveland, OH 44105. (800) 323-5513. Lumbar support cushions.

**Mead-Hatcher, Inc,** PO Box 861, Buffalo, NY 14240-0861. (800) 225-5644 or (716) 877-1185. Wrist and foot rests, above and below counter keyboard drawers, anti-glare filters, and other accessories.

**Nada Chair**, 783 N. E. Harding Street, Minneapolis, MN 55413. (612) 331-8018. Fax (612) 331-1613. Unique, relatively inexpensive back support sling.

**PC Compatibles**, 55 Valley View, PO Box 46, Chappaqua, NY 10514. (800) 487-0781. Footrests and various supports for the wrists and keyboard.

**Proformix, Inc,** 50 Tannery Road, Unit 8, Branchburg NJ 08876. (908) 534-6400. Negative slope keyboard trays, mouse trays.

**S. A. Richards Mfg** (Prop-It). (800) 722-6403. An inexpensive, collapsible book and document stand.

**Viking Acoustical Corp**, 21480 Heath Ave., Lakeville, MN 55044. (800) 328-8385. Fax (612) 469-4503. Footrests, wrist rests, keyboard stands, glare shields, task lights, and related items.

## Newsletters and Magazines

*CTDNews*, 10 Railroad Avenue, PO Box 239, Haverford, PA 19041-0239. (800) 554-4283. Industry-oriented newsletter published 10 times a year reporting on cumulative trauma disorders (includes noncomputer sources). Source for legal, insurance, and regulatory information. Cost is $125 a year.

*Managing Office Technology*, 1100 Superior Avenue, Cleveland, OH 44114-2543. (216) 696-7000. Fax (216) 696-7658. Monthly publication that covers the integration of technology and human resources in the workplace.

*Occupational Hazards Magazine*, 1100 Superior Avenue, Cleveland, OH 44144-2543. (216) 696-7000. Fax (216) 696-7658. Monthly publication that covers occupational safety, health, industrial hygiene, and environmental management. Subscriptions are automatically sent out to managers who purchase safety equipment through distributors. Paid subscriptions are $45 per year or $5 per copy.

*Occupational Health & Safety*, PO Box 2573, 225 N. New Road, Waco, TX 76702-2573. (817) 776-9000. Fax (817) 776-9018. Magazine focuses on practical approaches for business to comply with OSHA, Department of Labor, NIOSH, and other regulatory agencies guidelines, as well as information on voluntary guidelines, such as many ANSI standards. New products and new regulations are covered as well.

**VDT NEWS: The VDT Health and Safety Report**, PO Box 1799, Grand Central Station, New York, NY 10163. (212) 517-2802. Fax (212) 734-0316. Particularly well-edited, in-depth newsletter that covers electromagnetic radiation, ergonomics, CDTs, and other health issues related to VDTs. Annual product directory included in subscription. Cost is $127 a year ($150 outside the United States).

**Workplace Ergonomics**, PO Box 2573, 225 N. New Road, Waco, TX 76702-2573. (817) 776-9000. Fax (817) 776-9018. Ergonomic issues in industrial and office setting, focusing on practical means for compliance. New product and news sections. Slated to begin publication in October 1994; first regular bimonthly issue in January 1995.

**RSI Network Newsletter**. Grassroots electronic newsletter for people concerned about tendinitis, carpal tunnel syndrome, and other repetitive strain injuries. Available on many bulletin boards and on-line services. To subscribe via the Internet, send e-mail to: dadadata@world.std.com. Put "RSI Subscription" (without quotes) in the "Subject:" line and you will be added to the distribution list.

## Books and Pamphlets

**20/20: A Total Guide to Improving Your Vision and Preventing Eye Disease**, Mitchell H. Friedlaender and Stef Donev (Emmaus, Pennsylvania: Rodale Press, 1991).

**American National Standard for Human Factors Engineering of Visual Display Terminal Workstations**, Human Factors Society, Inc (see Organizations). Includes specifications of safe chair design. A new standard will be released in late 1994.

**The American Medical Association Guide To Prescription And Over-The-Counter Drugs**, Charles B. Clayman, editor (New York: Random House, 1988). Solid, comprehensive source for drug information.

**The Aspirin Handbook: A User's Guide to the Breakthrough Drug of the 90s**, Joe Graedon, Tom Ferguson, and Teresa Graedon (New York: Bantam Books, 1993). Everything you wanted to know (and more) about aspirin and similar pain relievers.

**Basic Stuff: A Survival Guide to Workers' Compensation**, Dorsey Hamilton. Compensation Alert, 843 2nd St., Santa Rosa, CA 95404. (707) 545-2266. $12 including shipping and handling, considered as a tax-deductible contribution. A worker-oriented guide to the California workers' compensation system.

***The Best in Medicine. How and Where to Find the Best Health Care Available***, Herbert J. Dietrich and Virginia H. Biddle (New York: Harmony Books, 1990 revised edition). Authoritative guide to top hospitals and specialty clinics in the United States. Includes rehabilitation clinics but not occupational-medicine clinics.

***Carpal Tunnel Syndrome: Evaluation, Treatment, and Prevention***, Mark Koniuch and John Palazzo (Thorofare, NJ: Slack Publishing, 1993).

***Employee Burnout: America's Newest Epidemic*** (phone survey conducted in 1991) and ***Employee Burnout: Causes and Cures***, Free pamphlet directed towards companies measuring organizational stress. Includes stress test. Write to: Northwestern National Life Insurance Company, PO Box 20, Route 6528, Minneapolis, MN 55440.

***The Ergonomics Payoff: Designing the Electronic Office***, Rani Lueder, editor (New York: Nichols Publishing Company, 1986).

***Get Well, Stay Well: The Successful Patient's Handbook***, Barry Gordon, M.D. (New York: Dembner Books, 1988). A blunt yet revealing aid for dealing with doctors and the medical system. Particularly insightful in the preparations you can make that help the doctor do the best job.

***The HAND Book***, Stephanie Brown. $19.95 plus shipping from: Ergonome, Inc 145 West 96th Street, New York, NY 10025. (212) 222-9600. Fax (212) 222-6699. Illustrated volume on hand and arm injury prevention from a pianist. Includes hand-positioning poster.

***Hard Facts about Soft Machines: The Ergonomics of Seating***, Rani Leuder and Kageyu Noro (Washington, D.C.: Taylor and Francis, 1993). (800) 821-8312. Professional review and assessment of current state of chair design. Expected to be published in August, 1994. Expected price: $99.50.

***Health Care USA***, Jean Carper (New York: Prentice Hall, 1987). Lists superior hospitals and health institutions in the United States.

***Healthy Computing: Risks and Remedies Every Computer User Needs To Know***, Ronald Harwin (New York: Amacom, 1992).

***Listen to Your Pain: The Active Person's Guide to Understanding, Identifying, and Treating Pain and Injury***, Ben E. Benjamin (New York: Viking Press, 1984).

***Promoting Health and Productivity in the Computerized Office: Models of Successful Ergonomic Interventions***, Editors Steven Sauter, Marvin Dainoff, and Michael Smith (London, New York: Taylor & Francis, 1990). Expensive, seminal work for experts.

***Repetitive Strain Injury: A Computer User's Guide***, Emil Pascarelli, MD, and Deborah Quilter (New York: John Wiley & Sons, 1994). Solid book by clinician with over 20 years experience treating CTDs.

***Sitting on the Job: How to Survive the Stresses of Sitting Down To Work***, Scott Donkin; contributing editor Joseph Sweere (Boston: Houghton Mifflin Company, 1989).

***Smart Questions To Ask Your Doctor***, Dorothy Leeds (New York: Harper Paperbacks, 1992). Useful compendium of questions to ask doctors to improve your chances of receiving the best care.

***Soft Tissue Pain and Disability*** (2nd ed.), Rene Cailliet (Philadelphia: F.A. Davis, 1988).

***Stretch and Strengthen***, Judy Alter (Boston: Houghton Mifflin, 1986).

***Stretching***, Bob Anderson (New York: Random House, 1980).

***Treat Your Own Back***, Robin McKenzie (Waikanae, New Zealand: Spinal Publications, 1988). Practical guide to back pain.

***Treat Your Own Neck***, Robin McKenzie (Waikanae, New Zealand: Spinal Publications, 1988). Practical guide to neck pain.

***The Wellness Book: The Comprehensive Guide to Maintaining Health and Treating Stress-Related Illness***, Herbert Benson, Eileen Stuart and associates at the Mind/Body Medical Institute of the New England Deaconess Hospital and Harvard Medical School (New York: Simon and Schuster, 1993).

***Workers' Compensation Claims Deskbook***, Gwen Hampton (Glendale, CA: Workers' Compensation Co., 1993). Referred to as the bible of workers' compensation, and reportedly used by caseworkers in California. $92.92. The latest edition came out August 1993. Workers' Compensation Company, PO Box 11448, Glendale, CA 91226. (818) 247-8224.

## Organizations

**9to5, National Association of Working Women**, 238 West Wisconsin Ave., Suite 700, Milwaukee, WI 53203-2308. (414) 274-0925. 9to5 is a membership organization run mostly by volunteers in local chapters. 9to5 focuses on protecting the rights of office workers. They have a job problem hotline—(800) 522-0925—for people to call who are experiencing or witnessing work-related problems of any kind.

**American Academy of Ophthalmology**, PO Box 7424, San Francisco, CA 94120-7424. (415) 561-8500. Primarily a support organization for ophthalmologists, individuals can call to get individual copies of brochures on health issues related to the eye.

**American Academy of Physical Medicine & Rehabilitation**, (312) 922-9366. Will supply names of physical medicine specialists in your area.

**American Board of Medical Specialties certification line**, (800) 776-2378. This nonprofit organization provides free information about doctors who are board-certified in a specialty, including the date that they were certified and for what specialty or specialties. (Except Alaska.)

**American Occupational Medical Association (AOMA)**, 2340 South Arlington Heights Rd., Arlington Heights, IL 60005. (708) 228-6850. Will supply names of occupational medicine specialists in your area. Contact Public Relations or Education.

**American Optometric Association**, 243 North Lindbergh Blvd., St. Louis, MO 63141. (314) 991-4100. They distribute a pamphlet called *VDT Users Guide to Better Vision*. They also certify glare filters and will tell you over the telephone which filters have met their certification standards.

**The Arthritis Foundation**, PO Box 19000, Atlanta, GA 30326. (800) 283-7800 or (404) 872-7100. Provides information and materials, including a free brochure on back care and back pain. In Canada: The Arthritis Society, National Office, 250 Bloor Street E., Suite 901, Toronto, Ontario M4W 3P2. (416) 967-1414. Fax (416) 967-7171.

**Association for Applied Psychophysiology and Biofeedback**, 10200 W. 44th Avenue, #304 Wheat Ridge, CO 80033-2840. (800) 477-8892. Local referrals for professionals who may specialize in CTDs and who incorporate biofeedback into their practices.

**Association for Repetitive Motion Syndrome (ARMS)**, PO Box 514, Santa Rosa, CA 95402-05124. (707) 571-0397. This nonprofit organization provides information on repetitive strain injuries. Publishes newsletter. They accept calls from 10 am to 5 pm Pacific Time only.

**Human Factors and Ergonomics Society**, PO Box 1369, Santa Monica, CA 90406-1369. (310) 394-1811. Fax (310) 394-2410. Worldwide professional organization for individuals working, studying, or writing standards in the field of ergonomics. They offer a directory of human factors and ergonomics consultants that is organized geographically and available for $35 to nonmembers or $20 to members. HFES also publishes papers including the ANSI standards on VDT workstations; a new version is expected in 1994.

**Illuminating Engineering Society of North America**, 120 Wall Street, 17th floor, New York, NY 10005. (212) 248-5000. Provides materials and referrals to local seminars and organizations to any size office on lighting. Publishes *Lighting for Offices Containing Computer Visual Display Terminals* (1989) for $35 plus $3 shipping.

**Job Accommodation Network**, 918 Chestnut Ridge Rd. Suite 1, PO Box 6080, Morgantown, WV 26506-6080. (800) 526-7234 or (800) ADA-WORK or (304) 293-7186. This free service of the President's Committee on Employment of People with Disabilities will supply information about the Americans with Disabilities Act to anyone who calls. The service which offers advice on how to accommodate the disabled is used primarily by employers, rehabilitation professionals, and by people with disabilities. In Canada, call a Canadian-government sponsored number: (800) 526-2262.

**Labor Occupational Health Program**, School of Public Health, University of California at Berkeley, 2515 Channing Way, 2nd Floor, Berkeley, CA 94720. (510) 642-5507. Nonprofit organization that provides job safety and health information, mainly to workers and the public. Maintains library and publishes educational material.

**National Headache Foundation**, 5252 N. Western Avenue, Chicago, Illinois 60625. (312) 878-7715. Nonprofit organization that provides general, up-to-date information about headaches. To receive information about treatments, send a self-addressed, business-sized envelope with 52¢ postage (in the US). Include a brief description of headache type and symptoms. A list of members in your state is also available on request.

**National Institute of Mental Health**, Office of Scientific Information, 5600 Fishers Lane, Parklawn Building, Room 7-103, Rockville, MD 20857. (301) 443-4513 (public inquiries branch). NIMH has free materials on mental health issues, including depression and psychological stress. They can't provide direct referral service, but they will refer people to professional organizations that can then provide a referral.

**National Institute of Occupational Safety and Health (NIOSH)**, Technical Information Branch, Mail Stop C19, 4676 Columbia Parkway, Cincinnati, OH 45226. Information line: (800) 356-4674. NIOSH offers a "help hazard evaluation" to qualifying employers, in which NIOSH goes into a worksite and evaluates ongoing conditions and then recommends changes, if necessary. Their report is given to the requester and to OSHA. NIOSH will also provide information about seeking local assistance in occupational health issues, but they do not refer people directly to other agencies or services.

**Office Technology Education Project**, 1 Summer Street, Somerville, MA 02143. (617) 776-2777. Nonprofit organization that provides training, education, and information about the health implications and the social impact of new technologies.

**Public Citizen Health Research Group**, Washington, DC. (202) 833-3000. Every two years Public Citizen updates a list (organized by state) of doctors who have been disciplined by state boards. You can order the section for your state for about $10. Public Citizen is a nonprofit organization that doesn't accept corporate or government money.

**Safety First Association**, 1400 Opus Place Suite 960, Downers Grove, IL 60515. (800) 432-4675. Fax (708) 963-3170. Nonprofit organization whose purpose is to coordinate a national testing service for ELF emissions from computer monitors and other equipment. Will refer you to various local and national vendors for internal radiation shield installation at discounted prices.

**TCO (The Swedish Confederation of Professional Employees)**, 150 N. Michigan Avenue, Suite 1200, Chicago, IL 60601-7594. (312) 781-6223. Fax (312) 346-0683. Certifies equipment meeting its ergonomic and radiation standard for desktop computers. Offers book explaining monitor facts ($27). Sells kits to help evaluate monitors ($10) and software ($100 with disk).

## Occupational Safety and Health Agencies

### United States
#### Information/Publications
Compliance with health and safety laws is administered either by a local or federal Occupational Safety and Health Administration (OSHA). To contact OSHA in locally administered states (or in Puerto Rico), call the local office; in federally administered programs, call the federal office. (See the regional office listing below to see whether your state is locally or federally administered.)

No matter what state you live in, for any OSHA publication, call your federal regional office. They will mail free publications directly to you. Some publications are available at a fee from the US Government Printing Office; the regional offices of OSHA will send you a catalog and other information on ordering paid publications.

Federal Regional OSHA Offices:

Region I: CT*, MA, ME, NH, RI, VT*. (617) 565-7164.
Region II: NJ, NY*, PR*, VI*. (212) 337-2378.
Region III: DC, DE, MD*, PA, VA*, WV. (215) 596-1201.
Region IV: AL, FL, GA, KY*, MS, NC*, SC*, TN*. (404) 347-3573.
Region V: IL, IN*, MI*, MN*, OH, WI. (312) 353-2220.
Region VI: AR, LA, NM*, OK, TX. (214) 767-4731.
Region VII: IA*, KS, MO, NE. (816) 426-5861.
Region VIII: CO, MT, ND, SD, UT*, WY*. (303) 844-3061.
Region IX: American Samoa, AZ*, CA*, Guam, HI*, NV*, Trust
             Territories of the Pacific. (415) 744-6670.
Region X: AK*, ID, OR*, WA*. (206) 553-5930.

States with an asterisk have locally legislated compliance. To call the local office, look in government pages in telephone book under "Occupational Safety and Health."

## Consultation Programs

OSHA funds free consultation programs that inspect worksites and advise employers on office safety. Contact the appropriate office in your state listed below.

| | |
|---|---|
| Alabama | (205) 348-3033 |
| Alaska | (907) 269-4939 |
| Arizona | (602) 542-5795 |
| Arkansas | (501) 682-4522 |
| California | (415) 703-4441 |
| Colorado | (303) 491-6151 |
| Connecticut | (203) 566-4550 |
| Delaware | (302) 577-3908 |
| District of Columbia | (202) 567-6339 |
| Florida | (904) 488-3044 |
| Georgia | (404) 894-8274 |
| Guam | (671) 646-9246 |
| Hawaii | (808) 586-9116 |
| Idaho | (208) 385-3283 |
| Illinois | (312) 814-2337 |
| Indiana | (317) 232-2688 |
| Iowa | (515) 281-5352 |
| Kansas | (913) 296-4386 |

| | |
|---|---|
| Kentucky | (502) 564-6895 |
| Louisiana | (504) 342-9601 |
| Maine | (207) 624-6460 |
| Maryland | (410) 333-4218 |
| Massachusetts | (617) 969-7177 |
| Michigan | (517) 335-8250 Health |
| | (517) 322-1814 Safety |
| Minnesota | (612) 297-2393 |
| Mississippi | (601) 987-3981 |
| Missouri | (314) 751-3403 |
| Montana | (406) 444-6418 |
| Nebraska | (402) 471-4717 |
| Nevada | (702) 486-5016 |
| New Hampshire | (603) 271-2024 |
| New Jersey | (609) 292-3923 |
| New Mexico | (505) 827-2877 |
| New York | (518) 457-2481 |
| North Carolina | (919) 733-2360 |
| North Dakota | (701) 221-5188 |
| Ohio | (614) 644-2631 |
| Oklahoma | (405) 528-1500 |
| Oregon | (503) 378-3272 |
| Pennsylvania | (800) 382-1241 (in Pennsylvania only) |
| | (412) 357-2396 |
| Puerto Rico | (809) 754-2171 |
| Rhode Island | (401) 277-2438 |
| South Carolina | (803) 734-9599 |
| South Dakota | (605) 688-4104 |
| Tennessee | (615) 741-7036 |
| Texas | (512) 440-3834 |
| Utah | (801) 530-6868 |
| Vermont | (802) 828-2765 |
| Virginia | (804) 786-8707 |
| Virgin Islands | (809) 772-1315 |
| Washington | (206) 956-5439 |
| West Virginia | (304) 348-7890 |
| Wisconsin | (608) 266-8579 Health |
| | (414) 521-5063 Safety |
| Wyoming | (307) 777-7786 |

## Canada

Canadian federal law mandates the existence of Workers' Compensation Boards in each of the 12 provinces and territories. The boards are essentially private companies which administer the workers' compensation program and provide educational services.

In some areas, the board also handles compliance for job safety and health regulations; in other areas, separate agencies deal with compliance and enforcement. Regardless of location, call your regional board community relations office (listed below) for information; they will refer you if necessary.

For publications and education, call the regional board. Some boards may provide printed material, while others can do on-site training, loan or sell videotapes or films, or refer you to organizations that provide this sort of training.

| | |
|---|---|
| Alberta | (403) 498-4900 |
| British Columbia | (604) 276-3141 |
| Manitoba | (204) 786-9667 |
| New Brunswick | (506) 632-2200 |
| Newfoundland | (709) 778-1225 |
| Northwest Territories | (403) 920-3898 |
| Nova Scotia | (902) 424-8336 |
| Ontario | (416) 927-3500 |
| Prince Edward Island | (902) 368-5688 |
| Saskatchewan | (306) 787-4370 |
| Québec | (514) 873-5828 |
| Yukon Territory | (403) 667-5224 |

## National Network of Libraries of Medicine

If you want to learn about a particular medical condition, these regional offices of the National Network of Libraries of Medicine will direct you to the most appropriate medical library in your area.

Region 1: DE, NJ, NY, PA. (212) 876-8763.
Region 2: AL, DC, FL, GA, MD, MS, NC, SC, TN, VA, WV,
    the Virgin Islands, and Puerto Rico. (410) 328-2855.
Region 3: IA, IL, IN, KY, MI, MN, ND, OH, SD, WI. (312) 996-2464.
Region 4: CO, KS, MO, NE, UT, WY. (402) 559-4326.
Region 5: AR, LA, NM, OK, TX. (713) 790-7053.
Region 6: AK, ID, MT, OR, WA. (206) 543-8262.
Region 7: AZ, CA, HI, NW, and Territories of the Pacific Basin.
    (310) 825-1200.
Region 8: CT, MA, ME, NH, RI, VT. (203) 679-4500.

## Committees for Occupational Safety and Health (COSHs)

For both union and nonunion workers who are looking for job safety information, the labor-supported Committees for Occupational Safety and Health (COSHs) are a good place to turn. Although labor unions provide funding and organization for these nonprofit and not-for-profit groups, you don't have to be a union member to get information and assistance from a COSH.

New COSHs are forming all the time, so for up-to-date information, check your white pages or business listings under COSH or contact a local labor union chapter, such as the AFL-CIO, or a state labor council or industrial safety and health council.

Although there is no formal national organization or structure for COSHs, the New York COSH (NYCOSH) is acting as a central source for coordinating materials and information. They also distribute books and manuals, although your local COSH may have these materials as well.

### COSHs
**Alaska.** Alaska Health Project, 1818 W. Norther Light Blvd., Anchorage, AK 99517. (907) 276-2864. Fax (907) 279-3089.

### California
San Francisco Labor Council, Fran Schriegberg, c/o Worksafe, 510 Harrison St., San Francisco, CA 94105. (415) 543-2699. Fax (415) 433-5077.

LACOSH, 600 South New Hampshire, Los Angeles, CA 90005. (213) 931-9000. Fax (213) 931-2255.

SA-COSH (Sacramento COSH), c/o Fire Fighters Local 522, 3101 Stockton St., Sacramento, CA 95820. (916) 442-4390. Fax (916) 446-3057.

SCCOSH (Santa Clara COSH), 760 N. 1st St., San Jose, CA 95112. (408) 998-4050. Fax (408) 998-4051.

**Connecticut**. ConnectiCOSH, 32 Grand St., Hartford, CT 06106. (203) 549-1877. Fax (203) 728-0287.

**District of Columbia.** Alice Hamilton Occupational Health Center, 410 Seventh St. SE, Washington, DC 20003. (202) 543-0005 (DC) or (301) 731-8530 (Maryland). Fax (202) 546-2331 (DC) or (301) 731-4142 (Maryland).

**Illinois.** CACOSH (Chicago Area COSH), 37 South Ashland, Chicago, IL 60607. (312) 666-1611. Fax (312) 243-0492.

**Maine.** Maine Labor Group on Health, Box V, August, ME 04330. (207) 622-7823. Fax (207) 622-3483.

### Massachusetts

MassCOSH, 555 Armory St., Boston, MA 02130. (617) 524-6686. Fax (617) 524-3508.

Western MassCOSH, 458 Bridge St., Springfield, MA 01103. (413) 731-0760. Fax (413) 732-1881.

**Michigan.** SEMCOSH (Southeast Michigan COSH), 2727 Second St., Detroit, MI 48206. (313) 961-3345. Fax (313) 961-3588.

**Minnesota.** MN-COSH (Minnesota COSH), c/o Lyle Krych M330, FMC Corp. Naval System Division, 4800 E. River Rd., Minneapolis, MN 55421. (612) 572-6997. Fax (612) 572-9826.

**New Hampshire.** NHCOSH (New Hampshire COSH), c/o NH AFL-CIO, 110 Sheep Davis Rd., Pembroke, NH 03275. (603) 226-0516. Fax (603) 225-7294.

### New York

ALCOSH (Alleghany COSH), 100 East Second St., Jameston, NY 14701. (716) 448-0720.

CNYCOSH (Central New York COSH), 615 W. Genessee St., Syracuse, NY 13204. (315) 471-6187. Fax (315) 422-6514.

ENYCOSH (Eastern New York), c/o Larry Rafferty, 121 Erie Rd., Schenectady, NY 12305. (518) 372-4308. Fax (518) 393-3040.

NYCOSH (New York COSH), 275 Seventh Ave., 8th Flr., New York, NY 10001. (212) 627-3900 (NYC) or (914) 939-5612 (Lower Hudson) or (516) 273-1234 (Long Island). Fax (212) 627-9812.

ROCOSH (Rochester COSH), 797 Elmwood Ave. #4, Rochester, NY 14620. (716) 244-0420.

WYNCOSH (Western New York COSH), 2495 Main St., Suite 438, Buffalo, NY 14214. (716) 833-5416. Fax (716) 833-7507.

**North Carolina.** NCOSH (North Carolina COSH), PO Box 2514, Durham, NC 27715. (919) 286-9249. Fax (919) 286-4857.

**Oregon.** c/o Dick Edgington, ICWU-Portland, 7440 SW 87 St., Portland, OR 97223. (503) 244-8429.

**Pennsylvania.** PhilaCOSH (Philadelphia COSH), 3001 Walnut St., 5th Flr., Philadelphia, PA 19104. (215) 386-7000. Fax (215) 386-3529.

**Rhode Island.** RICOSH (Rhode Island COSH), 741 Westminster St., Providence, RI 02903. (401) 751-2015.

**Tennessee.** TNCOSH (Tennessee COSH), 309 Whitecrest Dr., Maryville, TN 37801. (615) 983-7864.

**Texas.** TexCOSH (Texas COSH), c/o Karyl Dunson, 5735 Regina, Beaumont, TX 77706. (409) 898-1427.

**Washington.** WASHCOSH, 2800 First Ave., Room 208, Seattle, WA 98121. (206) 443-4721.

**Wisconsin.** WisCOSH (Wisconsin COSH), 734 N. 26th St., Milwaukee, WI 53230. (414) 342 1996 (ATU 998).

**Canada** (Ontario). WOSH (Windsor COSH), 547 Victoria Ave., Windsor, Ontario N9A 4N1. (519) 254-5157. Fax (519) 254-4192.

## COSH-Related Groups
**California.** Labor Occupational Health Program (See listing under Organizations).

**District of Columbia.** Workers Institute for Occupational Safety and Health, 1126-16th St. NW, Room 403, Washington, DC 20036. (202) 887-1980. Fax (202) 887-0191.

**Louisiana.** Labor Studies Program/LA Watch, Institute of Human Relations, Loyola University, Box 12, New Orleans, LA 70118. (504) 861-5830. Fax (504) 861-5833.

**New Jersey.** New Jersey Work Environmental Council, 452 E. Third St., Moorestown, NJ 08057. (609) 866-9405. Fax (609) 866-9708.

**New York.** Tompkins Courtland Labor Coalition, 109 W. State St., Ithaca, NY 14850. (607) 277-5670.

**Ohio.** Greater Cincinnati Occupational Health Center, 10475 Reading Rd., Cincinnati, OH 45241. (513) 769-0561 or (513) 769-0766.

**West Virginia.** Institute of Labor Studies, 710 Knapp Hall, West Virginia University, Morgantown, WV 26506. (304) 293-3323. Fax (304) 293-7163.

# Index

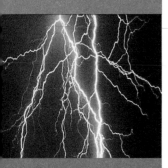

COSH. *See* Committee on Occupational Safety and Health
Counseling 87
CTD. *See* Cumulative trauma disorder
*CTDNews* viii, 137
CTS. *See* Carpal tunnel syndrome
Cubital tunnel syndrome 75
Cumulative trauma disorder (CTD) vii, viii, 59, 71–78, 79–83
   carpal tunnel syndrome 48, 73, 74, 75, 103, 108, 114, 124
   joints and 72–73
   medical intervention for 113–118
   and muscles 72
   and nerves 74–75
   symptoms 71–72
   and tendons 73–74
   treatment 115–116

## D

Danish clinical study 45
DataHand 64
Degaussing 29, 33, 35
Depression
   and drowsiness 95
   and headaches 19
   high-incidence jobs 85
   information on 87, 142
   medications 104
   stress and 84
De Quervain's disease 44, 49, 74
Dermatitis 84, 68–69, 91, 93
Desk 56–58
   adjustment 57
   conflict with chair 57
   height 56–57
Diet 95–96
   and antidepressants 101–102, 104
   and headaches 21
   and stress 86
Disks (spinal) 50, 79, 80, 81
DisplayMate 35, 127
Doctors ix, 114–115
   credentials and experience 76, 114–116, 118
   cumulative trauma disorders and 49, 76, 81, 113–118
   examinations 116–117, 118
   eye 10, 14–15
   headaches and 20, 21
   specialties 113–114
Document holders. *See* Copy stand
Double-crush syndrome 82
Double vision 8, 14

Drinking. *See* Alcohol
Drowsiness 95, 102, 103, 104
   from medication 102, 103, 104
Drugs
   illegal 86, 96
   legal. *See* Medications
Dry eyes 10, 11, 14, 16
Dual scanning. *See* Liquid crystal displays
Dust 32–33, 34, 91, 92, 93
Dvorak keyboard layout 62

## E

Elbow 67, 74
Electric blankets 42
Electric field. *See* Electromagnetic radiation
Electromagnetic field (EMF). *See* Electromagnetic radiation
Electromagnetic radiation (EMR) 36–43, 44–48
   avoiding 40, 69
   and cancer 38–39
   consultants 42
   electric field 34, 38
   extremely low frequency (ELF) 37
   magnetic field 38
   measuring 42
   MPRII 40, 48, 69
   from power lines 35, 36, 38, 39, 41
   and pregnancy 40, 44–48
   shields 34, 43, 132
   spectrum 37
   studies 38, 39, 44–48
   type from monitor 41
   very low frequency (VLF) 37
EK1 keyboard 67, 1XX
ELF (extremely low frequency) 37. *See also* Electromagnetic radiation
EMF (electromagnetic field). *See* Electromagnetic radiation
Emotional problems. *See* Stress (psychological)
Employee surveillance 87
EMR. *See* Electromagnetic radiation
Environmental Protection Agency (EPA) Energy Star program 40
Environmental engineers 42, 93
Epicondylitis 74. *See also* Cumulative trauma disorders
Epidemiology 38
Epilepsy 110
Ergoknowledge 112
Ergonomics 4
   ensuring workplace soundness 119–122
   training 121

## Q R

## S

## Permissions

Cartoon, page 3, ©1993 Nevin Berger, Laughing Trout. Originally appeared in *MacWeek* magazine. Illustration, page 19, adapted with permission of Charles Scribner's Sons, an imprint of Macmillan Publishing Company from *Migraine and Other Headaches* by James W. Lance, M.D. Copyright ©1975, 1986 Judith Lilian Lance. Illustration, page 50, adapted from a NASA graphic.

Photographs on pages iii, 4, 59, and 102, and keyboard detail on cover, courtesy of Apple Computer, Inc., photographer John Greenleigh for all but page 102; page 40, courtesy NoRad Corporation; pages 50, 55, 56, 58, and 68, courtesy Steelcase, Inc.; pages 63–64, courtesy respective manufacturers; page 79, courtesy Photo Stock; page 97, courtesy PhotoDisc; pages 110–112, courtesy respective software vendors.

## Keep in Touch

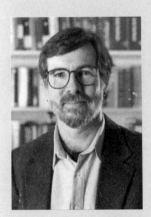

The computer-health field changes so rapidly that it's hard to stay current with the latest news and trends. One way to make sure I've got the complete and accurate information is to hear from you. Do you know of a super task light I omitted from **Where Else To Turn**? Have you found an effective treatment for a computer-related injury that I didn't cover? Do you think *Zap!* missed the boat somewhere? Or do you want to let me know I was right on course? I'd like to hear from you. Whether you want to discuss a product, a position, a story, some praise, or a complaint, please drop me a line.

Don Sellers
1619 Eighth Avenue North
Seattle, WA 98109

Fax: (206) 285-0308
CompuServe: 70421,3172
Internet: don@zap.com